Balance Exercises for Seniors

Prevent Falls, Improve Stability and Posture
with Simple Home Workouts

MICHAEL SMITH

Table of Contents

Introduction

"To keep the body in good health is a duty...otherwise we shall not be able to keep the mind strong and clear." – **Buddha**

Aging is a natural process. As we grow older, our bodies become more vulnerable to disease. There is no denying it; aging also dulls our reactions, slows down our movements, and keeps us from doing the basic things we used to do without any issues. But do we have to accept the effects of aging?

No, you don't; you can always fight back. The good news is that it is never too late to start exercising and getting fit. The earlier we start, the better it is for our health and well-being. Exercise is good for your health. It can help you stay fit and healthy, make you feel better, and even save your life. But what if you're a senior?

The benefits of exercise aren't about the cool abs younger people love to show off. It's all about the little things. It's about how your body feels when you're done with the day and when you start out in the morning. It's about how much energy you have in general and how much you have to spare after a walk to the supermarket. It's about what you look like in your clothes and how you carry yourself.

As we age, our bodies change—and not for the better. Our muscles start to atrophy and our bones become more brittle (they can break easier). Our metabolism slows down (we burn fewer calories) and our joints start to ache. The list goes on and on!

Exercise has many benefits for older adults, including:

- Improved strength, balance, and muscle tone. This helps prevent falls — a leading cause of injury among seniors — and improves overall health by strengthening bones and joints. Exercising is also an extremely effective defense against heart conditions, infections, muscle atrophy (muscle waste) and neurodegenerative conditions. It is a surefire way to reduce that extra weight; after all, obesity is a major cause of broken bones in older adults. Exercise also helps improve bone health.
- Increased energy levels. Improved circulation helps with blood pressure control. It increases the amount of oxygen delivered to cells throughout the body, which is especially important for older adults at risk of heart disease or stroke.
- Better mental health achieved through better sleep patterns and reduced stress levels caused by physical exertion (physical activity releases endorphins that create a sense of

well-being). Exercise can reduce symptoms associated with depression and anxiety disorders like dementia or Alzheimer's disease by increasing dopamine production in the brain. (Dopamine is a neurotransmitter involved in regulating emotions.)

And that's why exercise is mandatory as we age: you need it more than ever to keep yourself healthy and strong so you can continue to live normally. Even if you don't go on hikes or keep a garden, exercise is mandatory for everyone.

Exercise for seniors is important for more than the obvious reasons. It can help people with weak balance, those unable to move and go around their homes comfortably, unable to get up from chairs/beds on their own, while dealing with aging-related conditions like arthritis or diabetes. It's also beneficial for the mind and body to get in some physical activity, even if health conditions limit it.

For many, the question is, "is exercise safe for seniors? What if they have balance issues?" For many, balance can be a challenge. Whether because of age-related changes or other factors, staying on your feet and moving confidently is essential to living independently.

It's not that seniors do not *want* to exercise; it's just that they often *can't.* The truth is, people who have poor balance or balance-related issues face higher risks when exercising. The reason is twofold: one, when we're moving around and exercising, our bodies are constantly changing position and shifting weight, which can throw off our sense of balance. Two, regaining their balance is very difficult for people with weak muscles. So, even a normal sway to the side can turn into a fall. If you are just walking on the treadmill, an uncoordinated fall can lead to serious injuries like a pelvic fracture. Not only does our balance become worse with age, but our bones also become more fragile. So, even a minor fall can break the femur or pelvis. One out of every five falls causes an injury, such as a broken bone or a head injury. Each year, about 3 million older adults are treated in emergency departments for a fall injury.

So what can we do about it? First, don't worry—exercise can be safe at any age! You just have to be smart about what you do. There are a lot of safe exercises out there designed for people with balance issues. For example, many exercises don't require any equipment at all—they just require your normal body weight. So, there is no chance of falling off treadmills or injuring yourself from heavy weights.

Exercising doesn't mean that everyone should start running marathons or entering triathlons when they turn 60—it just means that if you've been sitting around watching TV on the couch every night after work all these years, try something new! It's never too late! Start by slowly increasing the amount of time you spend exercising each week. If you've never exercised before, start with five minutes a day and work up from there.

By moving more often throughout the day, you'll be able to prevent falls, one of the leading causes of injury among older adults. There are plenty of ways to get moving even if you're not a great walker or have trouble with stairs. In this book, we aim to show you just that. Based on research and experience, it is for people who have been struggling with their balance and want to get to the root of the problem. If you are tired of crutches and walkers or even need to sit when you cook and want to take control of your life, this book is for you.

The main theme is a safe and steady increase in balance and muscle strength. Balance isn't just about keeping your body upright—it's also about keeping your mind stable and making sure that you can always rely on yourself, no matter what happens. I want to help you achieve that.

The first step is to understand the cause. When you lose your balance, it means that your body is working with an impaired ability on some level. It's not always about the muscles, though. There could be something wrong with your joints, neuromuscular circuits, or even your inner ears. I won't tell you that if you do some exercises every day, this will all go away. It won't. If you have a serious condition that is seriously hampering your balance, you need to get medical treatment. If you suspect this, the most important thing to do is get checked out by a doctor or physical therapist. They'll be able to tell you if there's something wrong with your inner ear or spinal cord (which could be affecting your ability to keep yourself upright) or if there is another problem.

Most people find that there is nothing seriously wrong with them. Even if there is, you probably have a chronic condition like arthritis for which exercise can be very helpful. If, however, you find that your balance issues aren't due to a medical condition, it is still possible to regain your balance. You only need to work on strengthening your core muscles and improving your proprioception (the sense of where your body parts are relative to each other).

This weakens as our muscles grow weaker. But, what I have learned in all my years helping my father regain his balance is that muscles are buildable things. If you work out, your muscle fibers will increase in size and number. A new blood supply will provide for all muscles, and your body will start absorbing more nutrients to make up for the work they are doing. In short, when you put your muscles to work, your body will do its part to keep up with the new demands. All you have to do is increase the workload steadily and systematically to avoid getting hurt in the process.

The next step is to undertake a structured exercise routine designed specifically to improve balance. Programs designed by experts in this field have been proven effective time and time again. The good news is that they don't require hours at the gym; you can do them right at home!

When you do a balancing exercise, your body learns how to react with grace and poise. As with everything else, there is a correct way to do these exercises. It's not just about watching and following; that way, you never come to understand what you are doing and why. There are specific things to learn before you start so when you *do* an exercise, you understand its purpose perfectly.

We'll start by going over the basics: postures, the place, the equipment you'll need (or won't), how often you should be doing the exercises, and how long each session should last. Then we'll get into the good stuff—the exercises themselves!

You'll find everything from basic balancing techniques for daily purposes like walking and driving done easily as possible (and then some) all the way up to advanced moves like squatting and standing up, yoga, and moving heavy materials without assistance. We've got something for everyone, so join us and start moving toward better balance today!

****

FREE GIFT #1: FULL AUDIO-BOOK

Did you know that listening to an audiobook can help you retain more information? Enjoy the audiobook anywhere, without needing to carry a physical book. By listening, you can engage in physical activities at the same time, giving your eyes a rest from reading.

To give it a try, visit **bit.ly/Balance-audio** and grab the audio version (along with other free bonuses).

You can also scan the QR code with your phone camera if you prefer not to type. It's absolutely free.

I hope you find it helpful and enjoyable.

****

Chapter 1: Exercising as We Get Older

It sucks to get older. I'm not talking about the kind of older adult who spends all day sitting in a rocking chair, watching TV, and eating popcorn. I'm talking about the type of aging that makes your body ache, your joints hurt, and your bones feel like they're going to splinter into pieces any minute.

The thing is... I'm pretty sure this is exactly what is happening to you right now, just like it was happening to my mom and dad a few years ago. I can feel it coming for me too. As we grow older, our bodies change. We have different aches and pains, and it can be tough to keep up with the same physical activities we did when we were younger. It's a hard pill to swallow, but it's true, nonetheless.

We're certainly not saying that getting old is terrible! The senior years can be the very best years of your life if you can manage your health and battle the wave of loss of balance and muscle atrophy, and the pain that comes with it. In this book, I will show you how to do just that.

What happens to the body when you age?

You may not think much about age-related changes to your body, but as you get older, you experience them in different ways. One of the most noticeable is that muscle mass decreases. Our muscles contain cells called fibers that contract when we move. When we're younger, most of them are made up of fast-twitch muscle fibers, which contract quickly but tire easily. As we get older, however, there tend to be fewer fast-twitch fibers and more slow-twitch fibers in our muscles — which means we can't move as quickly or powerfully. However, this is only the start. After a while, all the types of muscle fibers start lowering in number. You can even notice muscle loss within the duration of a few months.

Your balance is affected by aging, too – especially as you age beyond 75 years old. Balance occurs when the brain and muscles work together to keep you upright while moving through space. When either of these systems breaks down or isn't functioning correctly, it can cause falls that can break bones or engender other traumatic injuries.

If this happens to someone over 70-75 years old, they are more likely to have a severe injury from a fall than those younger because their bones are more fragile, containing less calcium and bone-forming cells. So, they don't heal as quickly as younger people's bones. Falls also increase the risk of heart disease and stroke because they lead to injuries such as broken hips or collar bones that require surgery, which can be dangerous for elderly patients with other health issues such as high blood pressure. Not to mention, hip fracture repairs can lead to necrosis (rotting of the bone) if your body doesn't accept the prosthesis.

Clearly, all this can be avoided by having or regaining a good balance. Balance disorders can be either neurological or musculoskeletal in origin. In the first case, they are caused by damage to the inner ear or brain stem. These disorders include benign paroxysmal positional vertigo (BPPV), labyrinthitis, and vestibular neuronitis.

In the second case, they are caused by issues with the muscles that control balance or problems with posture. Balance disorders also occur from an injury or condition such as a concussion or stroke. However, most people develop balance problems later in life because of osteoporosis or arthritis in the joints such as the hips and knees, which results from wear and tear over time.

Training to regain balance?

The word "balance" is often used to describe the state of stability as we stand on two feet. But it is actually a complex process involving multiple systems in our body. When we talk about balance, we are referring to our ability to maintain an upright stance with minimal effort and remain steady in our current position, even when external forces act on us (e.g., bending down, going up the stairs, etc.).

Balance involves three mechanisms: regular standing, posture (keeping your body from swaying or falling over), and movement coordination (between your limbs and body). It also relies on eye-hand coordination as well as coordinated muscle contractions. Have you ever seen string puppets? Our balance is much like them; many strings need to work together for fluid and sure movements.

The question remains, is it possible to learn balance again? Especially at an old age? Actually, yes. In fact, the regaining process will help you both with your muscles and your brain. Learning indeed gets more complicated with age. However, the brain is like a muscle that needs exercise, just like the rest of the body. The more you use it, the more it grows. And with age, it tends to shrink.

But studies show that if you keep exercising and learning new exercises, you can slow down this process and even reverse some of the damage as you get older. That's why doctors recommend regular physical and mental activity for people in their 60s and beyond as it helps keep their minds sharp and protects against Alzheimer's disease and other memory problems that come with age. So, it's really a bonus!

Before you jump into the exercises, I recommend that you assess your balance first. It will give you an idea of what you are working with and how much you have improved over time. To test your balance at home, you need a stopwatch. To start, stand on one leg for 10 seconds and then switch to the other leg. Count how many times you can do that in 60 seconds.

Or, you can stand on one leg and see how long you can do it without toppling. Set a chair beside you for support so you don't injure yourself. If you can't balance for even one second, seek medical help immediately as it indicates a major problem with your nervous system or brain. A person with good balance can usually count on 2-4 switches of the legs during a 60-90-second period of time, while an individual with poor balance may not be able to do it at all!

What are the causes of losing balance so quickly? As I said earlier, there can be several causes. However, if you find that you can't balance on one leg for even 3-4 seconds, you should get checked as follows:

Medications: If you're on certain medications, such as antidepressants, antipsychotics, and beta blockers, they may cause dizziness.

Inner ear problems: Any kind of inner ear problem can result in imbalance and vertigo if you've experienced hearing loss or tinnitus (ringing in the ears), for example.

Heart disease: If you have heart disease or any form of cardiovascular disease (such as an irregular heartbeat), it could cause dizziness. The same goes if you have high blood pressure or high cholesterol levels; these are all risk factors for stroke, which can lead to dizziness.

Vision problems: If your vision is impaired due to age-related macular degeneration (AMD) or glaucoma, this can cause issues with balance, too; having blurred vision makes it harder to judge where objects are positioned, so you may lose your sense of balance more easily than someone with full eyesight.

Having any of these issues doesn't mean that you should not exercise. You absolutely should as exercise will help, especially if you have a heart condition. Remember, exercise and balance are more about the whole body.

The aging body and exercise

As we age, our bodies change. We know this. The brain shrinks with age, but exercise can prevent brain atrophy by boosting blood flow to the front and back of the brain. The heart weakens with age, but regular aerobic exercise strengthens the heart muscle. Muscles and bones lose mass as you get older too (even though they might not look it). Exercise can keep them strong. Blood vessels become less flexible over time, and the extra blood flow from exercise helps them become pliant. The skin becomes thinner and less elastic at the same time, making it harder for sweat glands to function properly when running or biking outdoors in hot weather because sweat evaporates more quickly than normal (and who wants that?).

It's true that cells become more fragile as we grow older, but studies show that exercising on a regular basis can prevent cellular aging as well. So, in the following chapters, we will learn about various exercises that target poor balance. The good news is that there are so many different types of exercises that can help you address your problems, no matter what they are. These are also home exercises that can change your life (and make you feel better than ever).

We won't get into the importance of exercise as we get older and how it can help us stay healthy and strong. We already know it. You will learn how to actually use the exercises. You'll also find out about some of the most beneficial exercises for seniors—exercises that help address common problems like arthritis and diabetes. Also, exercises for people with back pain and muscle gain (muscle loss also affects balance).

Why go into all the details? Well, as you get older, it becomes more difficult to maintain a healthy lifestyle. This is especially true for people struggling with chronic conditions like diabetes or heart disease. But there is some good news: by using these simple exercises, you can potentially build your balance again to a level where you can walk or even jog comfortably and get rid of the fall scares. And really, at this age, that's what people want.

For example, it's important to keep your vestibular system in good shape as you become older. This can help you avoid falls and injuries. But, most of us are rarely aware of it, let alone exercising it. For your information, the vestibular system is a structure in our ears made of two parts: the semi-circular canals and the otolith organs. The semi-circular canals are responsible for helping balance your body when moving around. They contain fluid and have three sections called semi-circular ducts. Each duct is filled with a different amount of fluid, which causes them to move in different directions depending upon how fast or slow you're moving. And based on these fluids, the otoliths help you detect gravity. Basically, they tell your brain whether or not you're upside down or right side up. They are made up of calcium carbonate crystals and very, very small hair-like nerves that move depending upon the position of your head relative to the ground.

If you are having balance problems due to vestibular health, there are exercises to restore it. Sometimes, medications don't help much, especially for age-related vestibular health decline.

Here are some exercises that can help:

- Tai chi is a form of martial art that uses slow movements to improve balance, flexibility, and strength. It's particularly good for people who want a low-impact workout. It works for your vestibular health with its flowing movements.

- Yoga can improve balance, flexibility, and strength. It's not as intense as tai chi but still has benefits if done properly.

- Dancing is another great way to improve your vestibular system.

- You can also try specific exercises targeted at vestibular health. This would probably be the best option. You can find these exercises in Chapter 7.

In later chapters, we will also learn about exercising for those with weak legs. After vestibular health, this is the most common cause of poor balance in seniors. We will also learn about exercises for the core muscles. We will discuss what exercises are best for each patient's personal balance problems (weak legs or core).

For those having trouble with their knees and ankles when they get up from a sitting position, an exercise that focuses on strengthening the outer side of your thighs and hips is recommended. This exercise improves balance in patients with weak knees or ankles because it strengthens all the muscles that keep you upright.

We also include a chapter on all the things you need to exercise. Don't worry; almost all the exercises mentioned in the book can be done equipment-free, but it's nice to step up and use certain pieces of equipment when you are ready.

So, there you have it. With a little work and persistence, you are set to start your balance-regaining journey. From there, you can go onto a strength-gaining journey as well, if you would like. I have another book on strength training over 40, so make sure to check it out.

If you are still confused about whether you really need to exercise or not, let me give you some more info. Regular exercise (exercise, not just walking) can reduce your risk of heart disease, stroke, type 2 diabetes, cancer, depression, and dementia. It also helps control your risk of developing high blood pressure or cholesterol problems. Regular physical activity will increase the amount of oxygen-rich blood flowing through your body tissues and the number of essential nutrients delivered to them as well.

You will also live longer and feel better. Many older adults struggle with depression and apathy. An active lifestyle reduces stress and improves mood in most older adults. This works on even the crabbiest seniors. Maybe you are struggling with post-menopausal mood swings or are just having a hard time dealing with the pains and soreness of joints. Taking up some form of exercise will really help.

Key takeaways:

1. With physical activity, you can maintain your body's strength and flexibility. This will keep you feeling good and able to do the things you enjoy.

2. Exercise is important for mental health because it allows you to feel happier and more positive about yourself.

3. Exercise reduces stress levels as well as increases energy levels throughout the day while reducing feelings of depression and anxiety!

Chapter 2: Get Set and Start

The first step of exercise? Sigh, shake your head, and mutter about how much you hate exercise. It's okay. We all do it. But what comes next is what truly matters. You crouch down on your mat and show the kids how to do it. You are still very much here and active, and you will build your body back and regain your mobility in no time.

If you feel apprehensive, don't worry. Exercise can be intimidating, especially if you're not used to it. But getting started is easy: just start moving. Next step: Get a doctor's OK. If you have any health problems — like heart disease, diabetes, or high blood pressure — talk with your physician before starting an exercise routine. Make sure you ask about any medications or conditions that might make exercise dangerous. After you have ensured that you are all fit to go, it's time to start knowing more and preparing yourself.

What to wear?

It may sound silly, but proper exercise gear is very important, especially when we don't want any falls. When getting ready to exercise, try to wear clothing that is both comfortable and easy to move in. Avoid wearing too much jewelry or other things that might get in the way of bodily movements. If you're going for a run, for example, it would be better to wear a T-shirt instead of a long-sleeved shirt because this will allow you more freedom of movement.

If you are exercising outside, make sure that your shoes fit, as they can affect how comfortable and safe exercising feels when walking or doing exercises on different surfaces like pavement or grassy areas. When putting on socks or shoes with laces, be careful not to tie them too tight as this could cause problems such as cramps in the calves (the muscles behind knees). Cramps cause pain during movement due to increased pressure against the arteries that supply blood flow through the leg veins back toward the heart. And finally, don't forget about sun protection!

Mental preparation for exercise

Prepare mentally for exercising before starting the actual exercises. Here are some tips:

- Set realistic goals for yourself and focus on your progress, not on how you compare to others.

- Decide beforehand what you will wear and bring it along so you can get ready quickly.

- Prepare yourself mentally by thinking about the exercise—what it is like, where it will be held, what the weather is like outside—and visualize yourself doing it before starting out on your journey (or even afterward).

- If you think of exercise as a chore, it will be harder to get started. Try to see exercise as an opportunity for renewal and relaxation or as a chance to meet people and socialize. Remind yourself that exercise has many proven benefits.

- Focus on the present. Try not to worry about how far you've come or have left until the end of your workout session (or your race). Instead, focus on what is happening right now—the music playing in your ears or the rhythmic thumping of your feet hitting the pavement as they move forward with each step.

- If possible, join an exercise group where you can share tips with other participants going through similar experiences; if this isn't possible for whatever reason, try at least talking about exercising with family members or friends who also enjoy doing it regularly–perhaps over dinner-time conversations!

Creating an area for exercise

First, let's be clear that this isn't an excuse to avoid exercise: it's an opportunity. It's so easy to let exercise fall to the wayside. After a long day at work, it's tempting to want to just plop on the couch and watch TV or scroll through your social media feeds. And you can, of course, but if you're trying to make a habit of exercise and regain your balance, one thing you can prepare ahead of time is finding space for it.

In our house, we have a small room previously used as a storage closet. It has since been cleared out and is now my home office. I cleared it out again, and it now serves as our gym too.

There are many ways to design a dedicated space for working out at home, whether you're trying to carve out a little corner in the basement or transform the living room into an oasis of sweat and grunts. The key is not to go overboard. Make sure to keep in mind how much space you really need (you probably don't need all that much), how much stuff you require, and how much money you're willing (or able) to spend.

Most of the workouts we will do are freehand and don't need instruments; all you really need is a yoga mat or any sturdy rug and an airy corner or individual room. You can also have a music player in the corner to give you an auditory boost!

Where and how to set up?

Choose a safe location. You want to exercise in a place where you won't be distracted by traffic or other people, and one where it's unlikely that you will fall. The gym is ideal because it has people around to help if something goes wrong, as well as mats and equipment specifically designed for older adults. However, they can be expensive and too crowded for some. In your own home, choose a location that's open, airy, and spacious. Also, somewhere not secluded so that someone can see what you're doing (and potentially offer assistance if you fall).

Some of the best places I've found include my backyard (if it doesn't snow when I'm using exercise equipment), my basement, or even the bathroom floor! Also, keep in mind that you want somewhere close by so it doesn't take much effort to get there when desired;

otherwise, motivation may wane over time due to a lack of interest.

Gaining flexibility and stretching

Stretching, warming up, and cooling down are crucial components of exercise. Plus, they increase flexibility, allowing you to move easily and naturally during everyday activities, like getting out of a chair or reaching for something on a high shelf.

Stretching prepares you for exercise by improving your muscle length and elasticity, as well as loosening tight muscles, so they're less prone to injury from sudden movements or intense activity. Stretching also improves circulation, which may reduce pain by increasing blood flow through the muscles being stretched. In addition, stretching helps prevent injury because it increases awareness of proper form while exercising (e.g., proper posture).

Stretching before working out prepares your body for movement; stretching after working out slows muscle fatigue, so you don't overdo it on subsequent days when performing similar activities such as exercise or daily chores.

Use proper form

One of the best things you can do to prevent injury and get the most out of your exercise routine, besides stretching, is to make sure that you're using the proper form. It's easy to assume since you've been doing something for years that there are no correct or incorrect ways of doing it. But whether we're talking about core exercise, yoga, or even walking around the block, there are always ways we can improve our technique to get more benefit from our workouts and spend less time in recovery.

In general, proper form involves keeping your spine straight with the shoulders pulled back and elbows by your sides. If possible, keep a neutral spinal alignment; don't let your back curve or flatten out, as this will put pressure on various ligaments and muscles, which could lead to injuries down the road if they become overstretched or chronically stressed.

Keep your feet flat against the floor when standing up. Avoid rolling forward onto the toes or heels, and don't let knees go past toes when squatting down. Also, don't rush your moves. Stay focused and slow. Slow and sure movements are the key to good balance.

Breathing during exercise

Let's talk about breathing now. As a general rule, the slower you are moving, the more important it is to breathe. Your rate of breathing should be regulated so you are not too winded, and your muscles can get a steady flow of oxygen.

A good rule of thumb is if you can keep talking to someone while exercising, you are good. Usually, this doesn't apply to all exercises; but, for beginners, it's a good rule.

Your breathing will increase during exercise because when you move faster and harder, your body needs more oxygen. If this happens too suddenly (for example, if you try to run up a steep hill without warming up), some people experience dizziness. You may also not be breathing deeply enough to fully expand your lungs; this is why abdominal or diaphragmatic breathing (also known as belly breathing) is recommended. Make sure to take normal, steady breaths during all forms of exercise and don't tuck your belly in and stop breathing to get more energy. You can hurt yourself.

Equipment you will need and cost analysis

For in-home exercises, you don't really need much equipment. However, it's still good to know the cost. It all depends on quality, brand, and availability. You can opt for low-cost items such as old sneakers or a mat from the dollar store or go all out with brand-name gear that will last for years. The choice is up to you.

First, before you do anything, choose equipment that's right for you. A pair of shoes that let you move freely will get you moving in no time, while a mat will cushion your body as you stretch and strengthen your muscles. A sports bra will keep everything where it should be during exercise, a good pair of shorts will be breezy to work out in, and a good pair of socks will prevent blisters that can stop any exciting fitness plan in its tracks.

Remember, your choice depends on what you are planning to do. If you want to go out every day and exercise in the park, pick a shoe designed for this. A sneaker designed for walking or everyday wear won't have enough protection or cushioning to protect you from impact if you're exercising actively, and it could even hurt your leg or make you imbalanced.

On the other hand, if you are exercising indoors, you don't really need running shoes. Before buying any type, try on a couple of different pairs before choosing one—you'll want to run around in the store a bit and see if any of them rub against your ankles or give you blisters. Do the same for mats too.

If you're looking for something to help improve your balance, look for texture, like a bumpy surface or grooves cut in the bottom. It might feel weird at first, but these mats will help make sure your feet stay planted while you're doing exercises that involve balancing on one leg. If you're looking for something more comfortable because of knee or joint pain, try a mat with a smooth surface. It'll be more forgiving under your joints as you move through poses and may prevent some of the stress that comes from standing for long periods of time. It might come with its own carrying case - great for storage when not in use. Some mats are "stickier" than others as they have surfaces that grip onto your hands or feet more tightly. This is really useful when you have a balance issue.

The material also matters. Rubber mats with extra cushioning can be quite expensive, but they're also more durable than their PVC counterparts and are known to last for years. PVC is easier to clean and less likely to smell after being used. If you're buying used equipment, make sure it is usable. Some people selling their old stuff might not realize that they can't get rid of the smell of sweat and bacteria.

After you have chosen your gear, determine the cost. Depending upon how serious you are about working out, you can spend anywhere from 50 to 500 dollars. However, don't go overboard! Just choose a good deal and start working out!

Key takeaways:

1. Preparation is getting the job half done.

2. Getting yourself mentally prepared and having all the equipment will help you start more firmly. You are more likely to stick to the schedule once you are committed.

Chapter 3: Exercise While You Sit!

Just as our bodies become used to a sedentary lifestyle, as we age, we find it harder and harder to pluck ourselves away from that inviting chair. If you've been feeling less than enthusiastic about exercise, then seated exercises are for you! They're only about 5-10 minutes long, but it is enough time to gain better balance. These exercises are easy to do at home with no equipment or at the gym on the seated rower machine. Even better, they can be done almost anywhere (assuming you have a supportive chair).

Despite what some may think, these exercises aren't just easy on the body, but they're easy on the mind too. There's something so gratifying about knowing that you're achieving something just by moving around in your chair! It's also comforting to know that exercising doesn't have to involve going to a gym or spending hours sweating over an elliptical machine; it can be as simple as using the muscles you already have available.

The best part? You don't need any sort of certification or training to do these exercises. They aren't complicated; there are no complex moves or techniques here! Seated exercises are some of the best ones to start for seniors. When you have been diagnosed with a physical disability or arthritis, it is best to start with seated exercises. You have less weight on your joints, which also helps relieve pain. Moreover, scientists have found that chair exercises can help you heal after a stroke.

Without further ado, let's dive into the suggested seated exercises.

1. Seated forward punch:

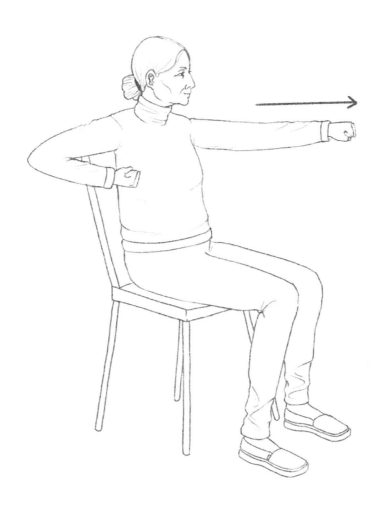

The seated forward punch is the core exercise for boxing. Its main function is to strengthen the body's shoulders, arms, and torso. Since it strengthens your upper body, it helps maintain the balance between upper and lower body. To gain balance, you need to match your lower body and upper body strength.

The way to do it is to sit straight on a chair or bench with your legs together; knees bent slightly. Hold both hands in front and close to your chest with the palms facing in and hands in a fist. Your elbows will be pointed outwards, and keep a distance of at least 4 inches between your elbows and the sides of your body while doing this exercise.

Position yourself so you can see a mirror in front of you. Ensure the back of your head and neck are relaxed throughout the exercise. Now, while keeping one arm in position - let's say left in this instance - stretch out the right arm as forward as far as you can while keeping them as straight as possible. Keep the right palm facing downward.

Now reverse this motion by raising your left arm and bringing the right arm back to your chest. Hold each position for 10 seconds. Then repeat this 8-10 times on alternating hands.

2. Pelvic tilt:

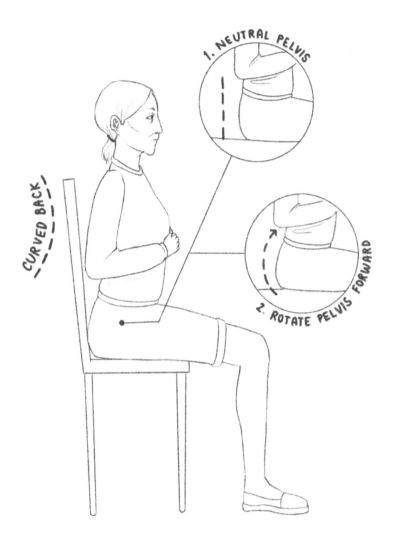

The seated pelvic tilt activates the muscles of your pelvic floor and abdomen; they are responsible for supporting your internal organs and keeping your spine straight. The exercise is performed by contracting these muscles (without holding your breath) while simultaneously relaxing the rest of your body.

Sit on a straight-backed chair with your feet on the ground. Now tilt your pelvis forward using only your abdominal muscles: you're trying to make your back concave with a little bit of your stomach sticking out. Try not to use any other muscle groups like the arms or legs. The tricky part is feeling these muscles working without an external reference point, but you'll figure it out in no time! Do 10-15 repetitions and 3 sets.

3. Seated toe raises:

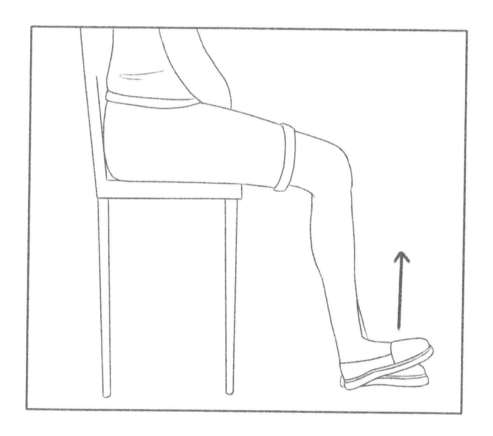

The seated toe raise is basically how you have imagines it: raising your toes. However, despite its simple name, it's a pretty effective exercise, especially for those with balance issues. To do the exercise, sit up straight with both feet on the ground. Flex your knees so that your toes are pointing toward the ceiling and hold that position for 5 seconds, alternating between feet. Repeat ten times. Those calf muscles will be burning before you know it!

4. Seated lateral flexion:

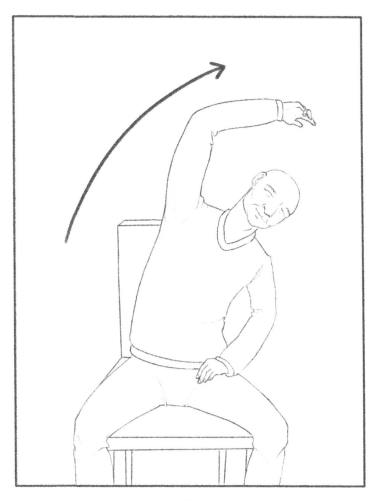

Lateral flexion is a movement that creates core strength in your back as well as mobility, effectively allowing you to strengthen your spine and neck muscles. To do this exercise, sit on a chair with back support and maintain a straight back. Put your right hand on your waist, holding the other arm straight up above your head. Slowly bring your raised left arm and your upper torso to the right side until you feel a stretch in the front of your shoulder. Hold for 5-10 seconds, then return to the starting position and repeat with the right arm in the air and leaning to the left side.

Seated exercises are the simplest and safest exercises to perform. Try the above-mentioned options in your home. Only after you have mastered at least three of them and can hold them for 6-8 seconds can you move on to the next chapter: standing exercises!

5. Seated forward bend:

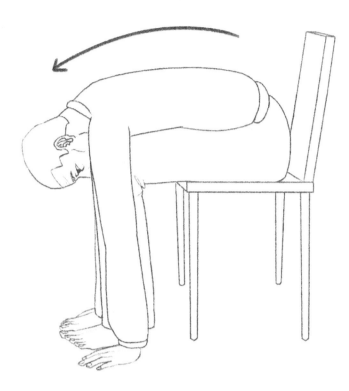

The seated forward bend is a simple and effective yoga pose, both for beginners and seasoned practitioners. No one should go all out too soon. In the seated position, sit up straight and take a deep breath in through the nose and out through the mouth. As you exhale, allow your head to tilt back slightly and your chin to drop toward the ground; you will feel a light stretch in the back of your neck.

Then reach your arms forward and try to touch the ground between your legs without moving your back. The spine should remain straight, and you should feel a gentle stretch in the hamstrings, thighs, and calves. If you find that it's too difficult to touch the ground with your hands, use a yoga block or two to prop your feet up until you've built enough muscle strength. This helps strengthen the back of the thighs and calf muscles, which are key for balance.

6. Seated hip flexion:

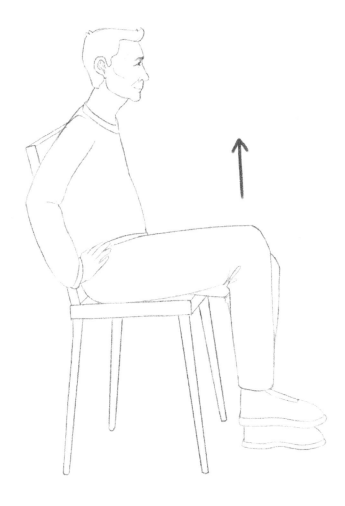

The seated hip flexion is highly recommended for seniors and those recovering from surgery, but it's also a great way to strengthen the muscles around your hips and lower back while improving your posture. To perform this exercise, sit on the edge of a chair or a bench with both feet on the ground, your back straight, and your abs engaged. Place your hands on the bench on either side of you in line with your shoulders. Or, if you are sitting on a chair, place your hands on your waist or grab the edge of the chair. Now, lift your right leg in front of you, keeping it in line with your torso and bending the knee. Hold it for 2-6 seconds, then do the same movement with the left leg.

7. Seated hip abduction:

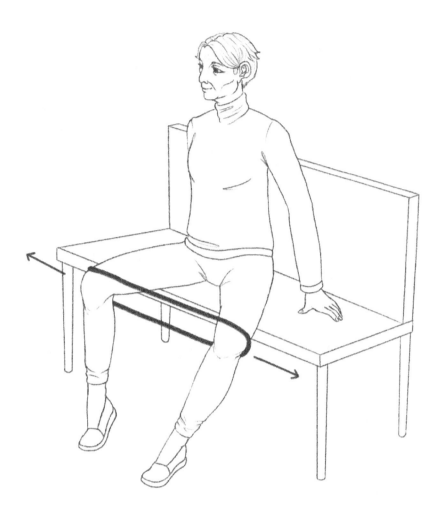

This is an easy exercise to do while sitting since you can use the chair and only the legs. You'll need a band made of rubber or fabric, available at most stores that sell exercise equipment. If you don't have a band, no worries! Use a stretchy clothing like shorts or T-shirt.

Sit straight in a chair. Wrap the band around your ankles or thighs. You can secure it with a knot or double it if it's too loose. Keep your feet on the floor with your knees slightly bent. Touch the ground with your full feet and wear shoes that make it easy to glide them. Plant your hand on the bench or the chair and move your legs apart as wide as you can without moving your upper body or back. You can move your hands along the legs too, but then you will need a back-supported chair. After you have kept the thighs apart for some time, pull them back together again as slowly as you can go.

8. Seated bicycles:

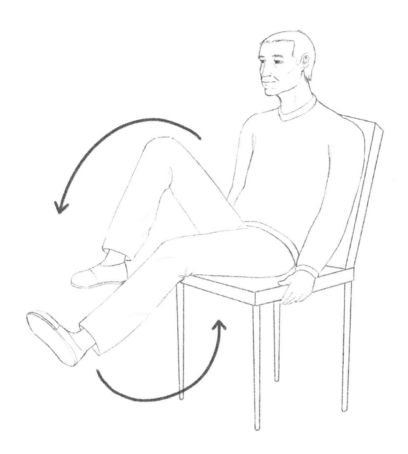

This one is a bit more advanced. Before you begin, make sure you maintain good posture and a strong back because this is the foundation on which all else will be built. Next, extend one of your legs out in front of you. Then, move it in an arc as if you are riding a bicycle. Lift your opposite leg and give the first one some rest. After you have done this a few times, lift both feet in the air and remember to pedal! While doing this, push on the armrest of the chair with your arms and back to increase your strength. Do the cycling for 1-2 minutes at first and then increase the time.

9. Seated hip external rotation:

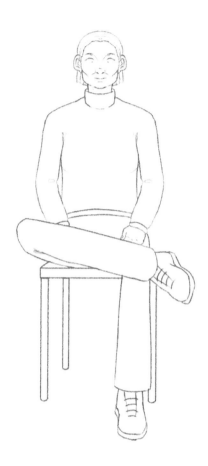

This will help stretch the muscles of your thighs and get some strength in them. To start, sit in a chair with back support. Keep both of your feet on the ground. Then put one leg over the opposite thigh. Keep your hands on your thighs and don't bend your torso. Keep this position for 3-6 seconds and then take rest for a few seconds and move on to the other leg. This is the basic form of hip rotation, but it's a good start for gaining fluidity in the joints.

Key takeaway:

1. When exercising, start from the easy and manageable ones.

2. Have a high backed chair without arm support for easy movement and more support.

Chapter 4: Standing Exercises

Standing exercises are a great way to stay active and build strength. They are especially beneficial for older adults who have balance problems, poor circulation, or arthritis. Standing exercises can also be useful for people who face difficulty getting up from the floor and need assistance getting back to their feet.

Some of the benefits of standing exercises are that they build strength in the legs, lower back, hips, ankles, and feet. This applies to older adults who may have lost some of their muscle mass due to age-related muscle wasting.

They also increase flexibility in the ankles, knees, and hips that helps reduce pain caused by arthritis or injury that affects these joints. Standing exercises improve balance by strengthening the spinal, leg, thigh, and lower back muscles so they can better support the body when standing upright. This helps prevent falls that could lead to serious injury or even death if you fall while doing something like walking around in your home or yard alone without someone nearby to help you get back up again quickly if you lose your balance.

The body's center of gravity shifts with age, so these types of movements are important for keeping the body aligned and balanced. Standing exercises can help seniors improve their balance, mobility, and strength. They can be done anywhere, anytime, and they don't require any special equipment.

Some of the best standing exercises for seniors are as follows:

1. Standing on one leg:

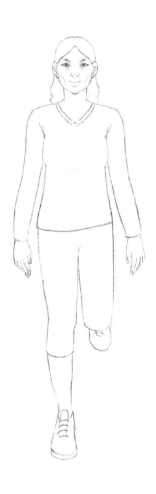

Stand on one leg and try to hold the position for as long as possible. Be sure to keep your eyes open and focus on something in front of you to avoid falling! This is an amazing way to build strength in your ankles, knees, and hips. It will also help you gain more balance since you have to maintain balance for a long time. Before doing this pose, keep a chair or a wall beside you for support and so you don't accidentally fall and injure yourself.

2. Single leg-arm stance:

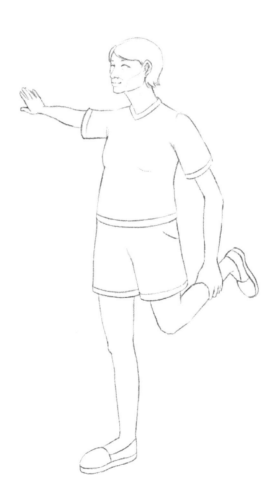

This exercise is a combination of the single-leg stance and the arm lift, which works your core muscles while building coordination and strength. It's also easy to do at home and can be incorporated into a warmup or cooldown routine.

For this exercise, start in a standing position, feet shoulder-width apart and knees unbent. Lift your right leg off the floor (only a bit high at first) and hold it at a 45-degree angle behind you. Simultaneously, raise your left arm above your head, parallel to the ground. Hold this pose for 10 seconds, then gently lower your foot and arm. Then repeat on the other side.

3. Rock the boat:

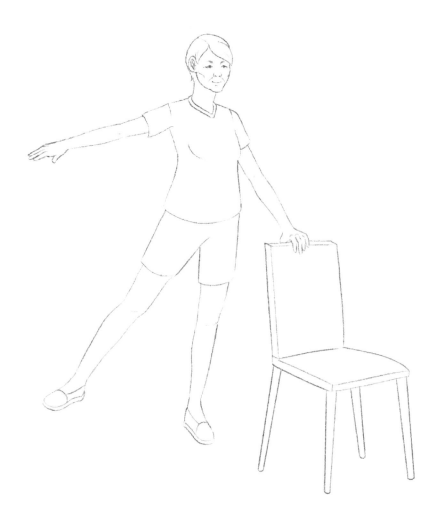

If you're experiencing anxiety or difficulty standing up straight, this exercise can help reinforce your balance and stability. Also, it will help you get your balance back. To perform this exercise, keep a chair or a wall beside you. Stand facing forward and gently lift your leg out to the side and move it slightly to the left. Now, keep this position for five seconds, then place your leg back down. Do the same with the other leg and repeat this on each leg ten times. After you have become comfortable, try moving your raised leg forward and backward in a rocking motion.

4. Heel lifts:

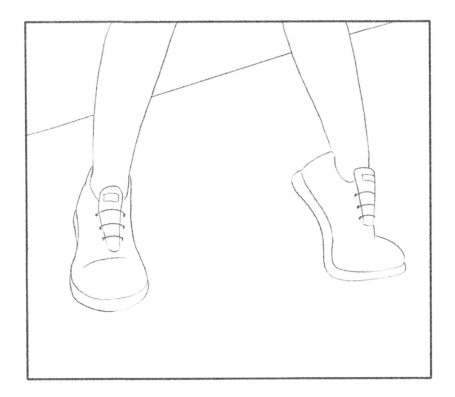

Heel lifts can be very helpful in stretching the muscles of your calves, which become flabby as we age. It will also help you gain a better footing. If you do them while standing behind a chair, it gives your body some extra stability and keeps you from getting as much fatigue or strain in your back.

To do this exercise, you'll need a chair. Stand behind the chair with both feet flat on the floor and slowly lift both heels off the ground while keeping your knees straight. Keep this position for a few seconds, then slowly move the heels back down to the floor so they rest flat against it before repeating the move ten times.

5. Balance beam:

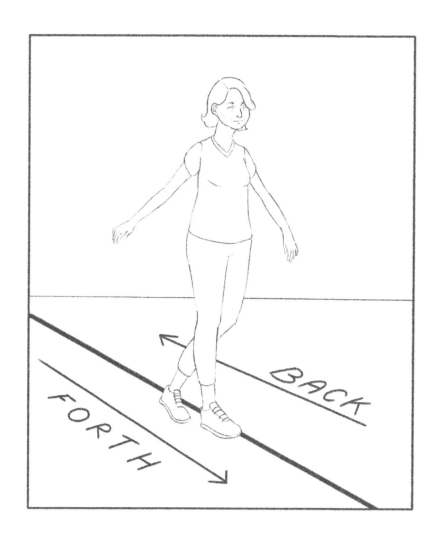

This balance exercise improves the sense of equilibrium. It exercises your inner sense of balance and your arm, leg, and torso coordination. While the original beam exercise requires a beam and is for gymnasts, mimicking that exercise by walking in a straight line on the floor is an efficient and easy exercise for seniors. This exercise will help build strength in both calf muscles and the core to help you regain balance.

You don't need any device for this exercise, but you will need your imagination. Imagine a straight line on which you are walking. Start with your heels on the ground and your toes pointed in the air. You can hold yourself upright by extending your arms or letting them hang by your sides as you slowly lift up one leg and move it forward. Then return to standing on both feet, again with your heel touching the toes.

6. Marching on spot:

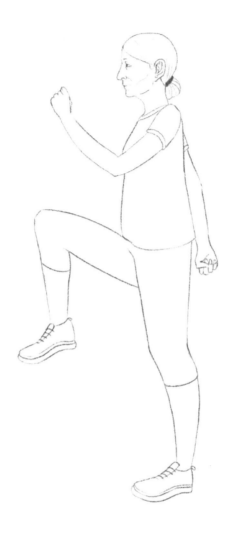

This is a very simple exercise; you can do it almost anywhere with no equipment. All you need is enough space to take several steps in one direction without bumping into anything (or anyone). To begin, face forwards. Lift your right knee and bring it towards your hip. At the same time, swing your left arm in front of you. Repeat on the other side and increase the speed until you're marching on the spot. Continue doing this at a pace you prefer for one minute (or longer if you'd like).

7. Side step walk:

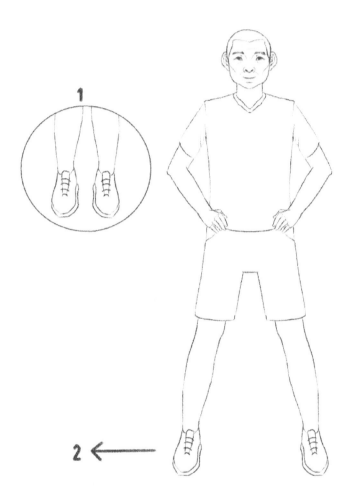

When you take the time to give your hips a little love and care, they will reward you with perfect balance. Just stand straight, facing forward. Sidestep out to your right with your right foot, then bring your left leg up. Move it to meet your right one. Repeat this for about 15-20 steps in each direction (forward and backward). You'll notice that this is a sideways movement instead of a forward or backward one. It allows you to focus on lateral movements, which are great for strengthening the hips and lower body in general. After you have mastered this move, try to jut out your hips a little bit and bend your knee while you sidestep. However, don't attempt this if you haven't regained good balance yet.

8. Stepping stones:

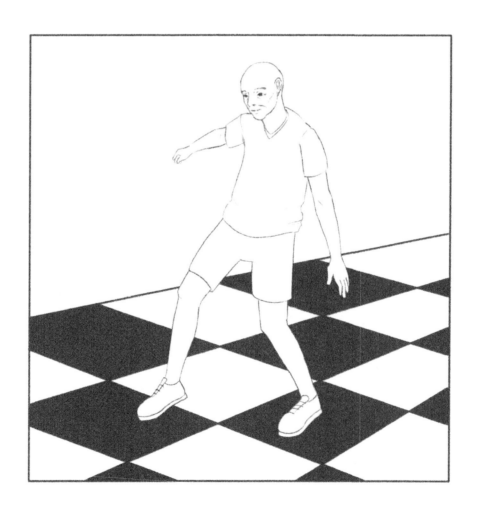

This is actually a game for kids but also doubles as good exercise for seniors. It will strengthen your lower extremities while working on balance and flexibility. To start, draw a few circles in an uneven pattern. You can use round rugs as well. If you don't have a mat handy or are pressed for time, do this on your living room patterned floor.

Begin by stepping into a circle with your right leg. This circle can be the size of a rug or a step—the size doesn't matter. The important thing is to step into the circle with your right foot. As you do this, take a deep breath and exhale as you step to the center of the circle with your left foot. Continue taking deep breaths as you move from one circle to another, using your right foot to enter each one before stepping fully into the center.

Key takeaways:

1. You don't have to be able to walk fast or have a high muscle mass to gain balance.

2. The small muscles you use while walking (the muscles that enable you to raise your knees and toes, turn your feet outward, and flex your ankle) also help stabilize you when

standing. So, exercising them will help you gain better balance.

3. To stand with good balance, keep your weight evenly distributed over both legs to gain balance.

4. The more balancing exercises you practice, the better you will get.

Chapter 5: Walking Exercises

Walking is an important part of any healthy lifestyle, but it does a lot more than just help you stay in shape. It's a great way to prevent falls as well as give your body better balance and coordination, so you can be more agile in your day-to-day life. Walking exercises are a great way to improve overall fitness while also helping you maintain or even improve your strength, endurance, flexibility, and mobility. These types of exercises are done everywhere at any time and keep you active without the need for special equipment.

Moreover, walking exercises for seniors are a great way to help them regain balance and mobility after being injured, having a stroke, or when suffering from Parkinson's. Many times, simple balancing exercises can lead to as much improvement as surgery or medication, but with less risk and a smaller chance of complications. Though experts in the field recommend regular exercise as the best way to combat the effects of aging and infirmity, many studies have shown that even short bouts of activity can help spur further recovery in patients who have limited mobility due to age or injury.

A walking exercise is basically any type of walking in which you're doing more than just going from Point A to Point B. You may already practice some walking exercises if you are working or going out each day. But even if you don't do these activities, there are several ways to get creative and increase your balance. Let's dive into some easy-to-do walking exercises for you.

1. Heel to toe walk:

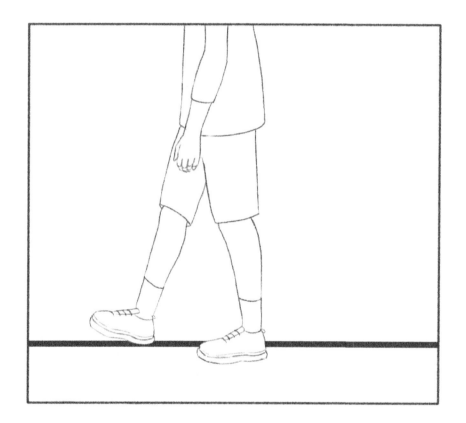

We did the standing version in a small capacity in the last chapter. Now let's take this to the next level. Walking heel-to-toe forces you to pay attention to every step, and you have to be mindful of every movement. Start from the heel-to-toe position, with your arms stretched out from your sides for support. Walk forward in a heel-to-toe fashion as if you are following black lines on a white floor. This means that you place the heel of one foot directly in front of the toe of the other as if you were drawing a line with each step.

Do this for 2-3 minutes on an even ground. Try this exercise in your backyard or front yard, and after a while, you will have better balance.

2. Balance walk:

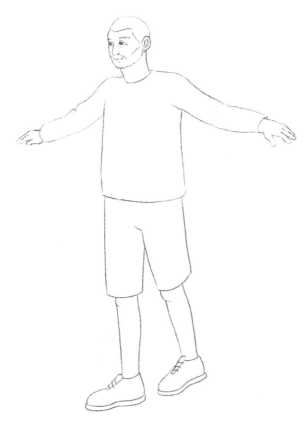

Balance walking is a great exercise for increasing stability, especially for those who have suffered an injury or are recovering from a fall and are afraid to start again. It can also be a good way to maintain balance among the elderly. Balance walking is done by walking slowly and deliberately, with a focus on keeping your upper body stable and moving forward at all times.

Start by focusing on keeping your head steady and looking at a fixed point straight ahead of you while you take very small steps to keep your feet in the same place. You shouldn't move your upper body much nor lower your hands. If anything, try to imagine that you're standing with your arms at your sides, palms flat, and pointing out. But continue walking forward in small measured steps.

3. Zigzag walk:

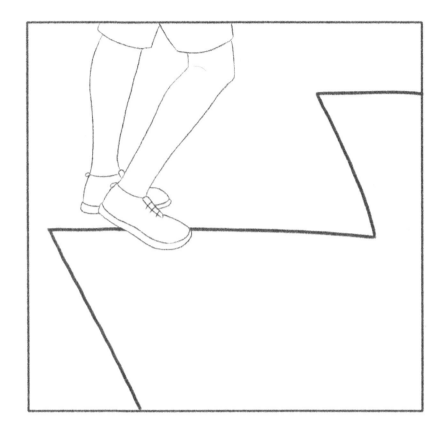

As the name suggests, the zigzag walk is a series of alternating steps. The goal is to keep your balance on the balls of your feet while making a smooth transition from side to side. It looks like a dance move, but it's actually a very functional exercise for the lower body.

To do this exercise, walk towards your right for 2-3 steps and switch to the other way for three steps. Go back to the first way for three steps, then switch again for three more steps. Do this several times. You can also draw a zigzag line on the driveway or pavement and follow the lines.

It may seem easy at first, but it does get harder—after even a few tries. You'll probably find yourself slightly off-kilter. The more you practice this walking exercise, however, the stronger your balance will become.

4. High knee walk:

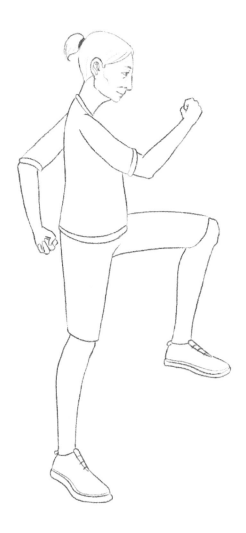

Walking with knee lifts gives your body a new way to adjust the limbs in addition to strengthening your leg muscles; the movement works your core, too. It is also a good way to practice balancing. To do this exercise, start with your feet shoulder-width apart, facing forward with your hands at your sides. Lift one knee until it's parallel to the ground, then lower it back down without letting the foot touch the ground. Repeat with the other knee for one to three sets. Also, lift your opposite forearms with your knees. Now, start walking forward while lifting the knee each time you take a step. Keep the steps small and slow so that you don't fall.

Also, make sure that you're lifting both knees as evenly as possible—if you're leaning to one side at a time, it'll throw off your balance.

5. Grapevine

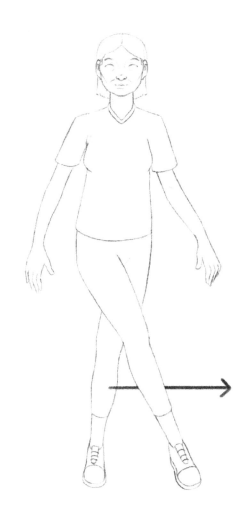

This exercise is beneficial to nearly everyone since it helps strengthen your balance and coordination, which are key in avoiding falls and also in preventing injury as you age. Start by standing with your feet together or apart and facing in one direction. Move one foot behind you and place it flat on the floor. Then bring your other foot over and to the side, let's say your right, and place it securely. Now, move the first foot forward and place it to your right. Repeat this movement in a slow, controlled manner ten times on each side.

6. Step up:

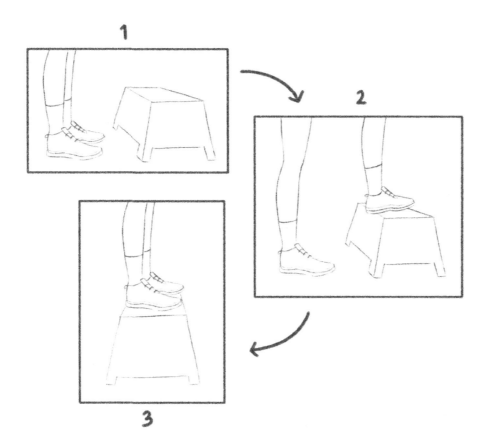

Step-ups are a great way to test your balance and strengthen your legs and back. In case you haven't seen them before, step-ups involve standing on an object (like a sturdy step or even a couple of books) and stepping up onto the platform with one foot and then the other.

Stand with your hands on the step for support and begin lifting one foot off the ground. Lift it just high enough such that you still have contact between your foot and the ground if you were to let go of the step, but not so high that your foot would be in danger of hitting the ground if you were suddenly pushed away from it. Bend your knee slightly to help keep your balance.

Step up onto the step with your other foot while keeping the lifted foot planted on the ground. Slowly raise that foot as well. Now, place both feet securely on the step. Now, it's time to step down. Step back down with one leg after another, so you're back on both feet again. Try not to lean too much or put your weight on either leg when you're standing still. Subtly shift your weight back and forth between both feet while you step up and down.

In sum, walking is a great exercise for improving balance and helping you develop a sense of your own center of gravity. In this chapter, we discussed how to do it well to regain your balance and health. The last piece of advice is to focus on your posture. The process affected by how tall you are, but it also depends upon your shoulders and torso, hunching habits, the back when you're standing up straight...and so on. The biggest mistake is walking around with a poor posture when you are prone to falling. To improve your posture, just follow a few tricks:

1. Look ahead with your chin tucked/or level with the ground.

2. Your shoulders should be back. Try practicing lowering your shoulder while walking.

3. Don't put pressure on your spine; just stand comfortably.

Key takeaways:

1. The smaller the steps, the less likely a stumble or fall will occur. So, take it easy and concentrate on the exercises while walking.

2. Posture is the position of your body in relation to gravity. Try making sure you have a good one to prevent falls.

Chapter 6: Core Exercises

The core is the center of strength in the body that supports posture, balance, and overall well-being. Different muscle groups work together to help you perform everyday tasks, like standing, walking, and bending down to pick things up. Whenever you do these movements, you're using your core muscles.

To recap, the core is a collection of muscles in the center of the body that work together to keep you upright and balanced. It's a complex network that also plays a role in other actions. The core includes muscles in the hips, chest, and lower back that work together to keep your spine and torso moving as one unit. In this way, you can bend forward at the waist easily without arching your back too much or tipping over on your heels. When these muscles are all working together, it helps achieve a proper posture and keeps you from experiencing back pain or lower back strain.

That said, some exercises focus specifically on strengthening these critical muscles and improving their overall function. Often, we mistake these abdominal workouts and the resistant training done at the gym by young people as mere aesthetics. They are really not; neither are they just for the young. Core strength helps reduce the risk of injuries and falls. Researchers, in fact, suggest them more to older adults than youngsters. According to research, exercise can treat osteo sarcopenia, reduce inflammation and rheumatoid arthritis, prevent falls, and even fight aging. All this is done specifically for older adults, so there is no reason why you can't start core exercises too.

The core muscles are situated at the center of gravity of the body. Imagine a structure or building; it is only as strong as the foundation beams running through it. It's the same for people. When you have a solid core, your body works as one solid unit, and it's very difficult to topple over. So without further ado, here are three of my favorite exercises that should help you improve your balance! Just make sure to master the exercises of the previous chapters for at least a month before attempting these. You don't want to rush it!

1. Abdominal crunches:

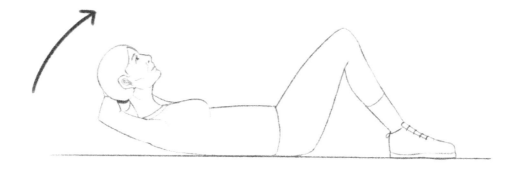

Abdominal crunches are a specific type of core exercise. Crunches work the rectus abdominis muscle, located in the front of the abdomen. This is one of the most popular core exercises for seniors as it can be done lying down without the risk of falling.

To do this exercise, start by lying down position on the floor and bending your knees with your feet planted on the ground. Have someone spot you (hold down your feet). Put your hands up and behind your head and lift your shoulders off the floor. Your spine should be straight and your back in a neutral position. Exhale as you contract your abdominals to curl forward. The forearms should be placed perpendicular to the floor at all times during the movement. Inhale while returning to the starting position.

2. Single leg lift:

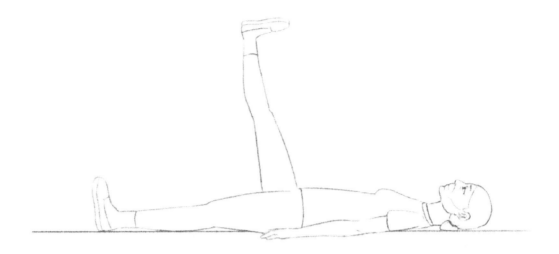

Single leg lifts are a great beginner's exercise, and one of my favorite ways to warm up before a core workout. A single leg lift is a great exercise to work your core, lower body, arms, and upper back. Lie flat and keep your arms and legs extended, palms on the floor or facing you as the starting position for the exercise. Blow out air from your lungs and tighten your abs. Your glutes should be tight, too.

Slowly raise one foot off the floor, keeping it straight, using the ball of your foot to push yourself off the floor. Keep your free leg relaxed and straight on the ground; try and keep it as still as possible. You can use your arm or the opposite leg for support if needed. Hold this position for 10 seconds. Now lower one leg back to the ground and repeat with your other leg.

3. Seated leg lifts:

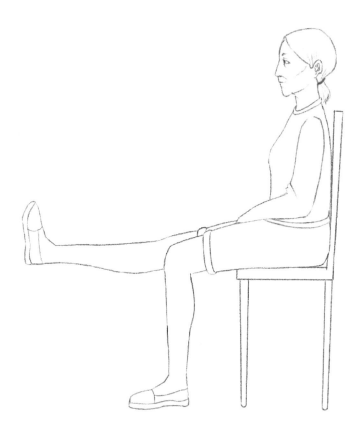

Seated leg lifts are good for toning the lower abdominals. Sit in a firm chair with bent knees, back straight, and feet placed firmly flat on the floor. Keep your arms beside your body, or keep them straight. Now, lift one leg off the ground making sure you keep the leg straight. Lift it to hip level and slowly lower it back down again.

Do this ten times, and then switch legs.

Ensure that your feet are pointed straight ahead; your legs should remain straight during each repetition. This is a very simple exercise, but it will effectively strengthen the muscles you use when climbing stairs, getting up, or walking. This can also be a great exercise to do with a partner or groups—it's great for bonding. Since it doesn't require any equipment, you can do this anywhere and at any time.

4. Modified plank:

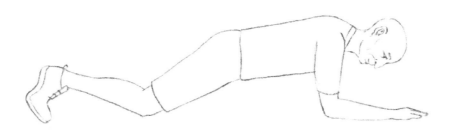

Before moving on to the standard plank, try this version on your knees. This is easier than the regular plank but has many similar benefits. Modified planks using your knees help strengthen your upper body, torso, and back muscles. As you are not putting all your weight on your feet, there is less chance of injury as well.

To do this exercise, start in a pushup position, your hands directly under your shoulders, then lower yourself to the ground on your knees. Your upper body should be straight and parallel to the floor. Your butt will be off the ground with only your toes touching it. Keep this position for 5-6 seconds at first and increase up to 30 seconds if you can. Do it against a desk if the exercise seems difficult to do on the ground.

5. Modified push-up:

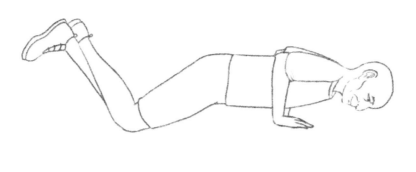

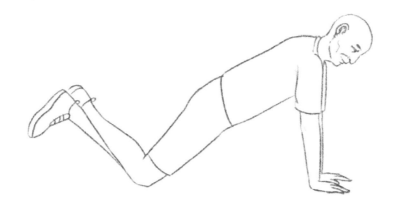

Modified pushups are an easier version of a push up that doesn't put stress on your body as much. There are several modifications; you can choose the ones you feel most comfortable with.

You can :

- Use your knees instead of your feet to put your body weight on.

- Place your hands on a lower surface, such as a bed or couch.

- Use a higher surface, like a desk or countertop, to push up against.

- You can also try doing pushups against a wall at first.

To start, put your hand on a surface of your choice and get into the plank position. Bend your elbows to lower your face and upper body and go as low as you can. Then straighten your elbows again. Do this 2-3 times at first.

6. Seated knee tucks:

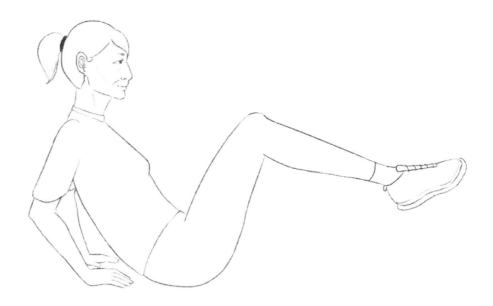

The seated knee tuck is a great exercise to strengthen your core and strengthen your legs, and thighs. It will help you exercise the muscles of the back of the legs, and it is for abdominal muscles coordination. Start by sitting on the floor with your knees bent and feet flat on the ground or on a mat.

Next, engage your abdominal muscles so your spine stays straight; avoid arching or leaning forward. Now, raise both of your legs and keep the knee bent. Then push both your legs forward as straight as you can, but don't touch the ground. Try to keep your back as straight as possible, but don't worry if that's not possible at first. If you can't lift all the way up at first, that's okay! Just try to get higher every day. Eventually, you will be able to lift yourself up all the way without help from your hands.

7. Plank:

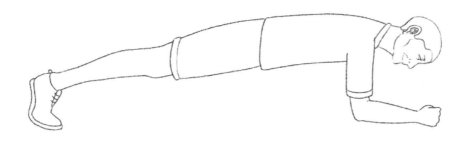

Planks are another good core exercise for seniors. Planks work your entire abdominal region, including your obliques, transversus abdominis, and rectus abdominis. Start on all fours (hands and knees). Then straighten your legs and lift up onto your toes, and balance on your elbows. The forearms should be flat on the floor. You need to keep your back straight and core tight while supporting your weight on your forearms and toes. Don't let your hips sag or raise up too high. You will form a single straight line from head to toe. Breathe in from your nose and breathe out through your mouth as you engage in slow and steady breathing.

Doing planks is difficult at first. So, take them slowly and start with the modified version.

8. Mountain climber:

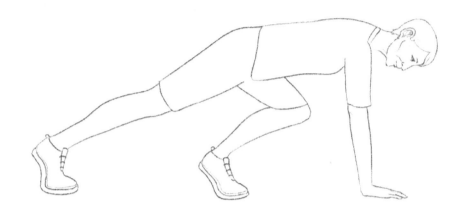

The mountain climber exercise is a high-intensity exercise that targets the quadriceps, hamstrings, glutes, and calves. It also works your core for stability. To start, get into a plank position. Keep your arms straight like you would do if you were to do pushups. Lift your knees and hips so only your toes and palms touch the ground. Squeeze your butt and engage your quads so you're lifting up from the floor rather than sinking into it.

Now, bring one knee toward your chest while keeping your toes on the ground. Then straighten this leg and pull up the other knee. Do this a few times until you get the hang of it.

Before doing any of these exercises, make sure to warm up. Start with a few gentle stretches to get the blood flowing through your muscles. Don't push yourself too hard—save it for the main workout! Stretching can help get the blood flowing to your muscles, which in turn makes them more pliable and less susceptible to muscle spasms and injury. Stretch before *and after* core exercises.

MAKE A DIFFERENCE WITH YOUR REVIEW

"Helping one person might not change the whole world, but it could change the world for one person." - **Unknown**

People who give selflessly often find joy in the smallest of gestures. It's in this spirit of kindness and generosity that I ask for a small favor from you.

Would you be willing to extend a helping hand to someone you've never met, with no expectation of recognition?

Who is this person, you wonder? They're a lot like you, or perhaps how you once were. They're eager to learn, improve their health, and regain the core strength of their youth, but they're unsure where to start.

My mission is to make exercises for seniors something everyone can enjoy and benefit from. To achieve this, I need to reach as many people as possible.

That's where you come in. Most people rely on reviews when choosing a book, so here's my request on behalf of a senior citizen you've never met:

Please take a moment to leave a review for this book.

Your review, which takes less than 60 seconds to write, won't cost you a thing, but it could profoundly impact another senior's life. Your words could help...

...one more grandparent play with their grandkids without pain.

...one more retiree enjoy their golden years to the fullest.

...one more neighbor participate in community activities.

...one more friend share smiles and stories without discomfort.

...one more dream of a healthy, active life come true.

To spread this joy and make a real difference, simply leave your review on Amazon by going to this link: **amzn.to/3T1Q6zp**

Or scan QR code with your camera:

If the thought of helping a fellow senior citizen brings a smile to your face, you're exactly the kind of person I cherish.

Thank you from the bottom of my heart. Let's get back to our journey towards better health and happiness.

Your biggest fan, Michael Smith

PS - Remember, sharing knowledge is one of the best ways to show you care. If you believe this book can help another senior, don't hesitate to pass it along. Your recommendation could be the start of their journey to a healthier, happier life.

Chapter 7: Vestibular Exercises

The vestibular organ is one of your body's most important sensory organs. It is located in your inner ear and is responsible for hearing, equilibrium, and balance. As part of your ear, it contains fluid-filled tubes called semicircular canals, shaped like half circles. This fluid moves when you move your head; and when they move in response to motion or head-turning (as when you're walking), they cause pressure changes. This stimulates nerve signals to travel from these organs up into the brainstem, where they provide information about movement and spatial orientation—information that helps control our posture and movements, so we don't fall over when we walk downstairs, etc.

The three semicircular canals within the vestibular organ help you keep your balance by sensing changes in rotational movement (that is, moving left or right). They also detect head tilts and movements that occur when you look down at the ground or up at something high above you.

The inner ear also has two otolith organs that use gravity to determine if you're upright or upside down. Together with other parts of the inner ear, such as cochlear structures (which are responsible for hearing), these five components make up what we commonly refer to as "balance."

Vestibular exercises are really a way to recalibrate the vestibular organs. They help seniors with dizziness and poor balance. The exercises are easy for seniors and their loved ones to do, and they can be done in the comfort of your own home. For those who have dizziness issues, vestibular exercise can improve their ability to walk without falling or feeling faint. It also improves their awareness of what's going on around them while they're walking.

Balance exercises can be very effective at helping seniors stay upright on their feet without falling over onto the ground or having to lean into furniture while standing up. These simple movements not only help improve balance but also prevent falls which may result in serious injuries such as broken bones or internal bleeding that could require surgery if left untreated!

The vestibular system is responsible for certain body movements like eye movements and head-turning, as well as balance control. When you move around in space, your eyes have to work together with your brain so they can keep track of where objects are located in relation to each other. For example: If someone walked across a room while talking on their cell phone without looking at where they were going—or if they spun around quickly—they would likely lose their balance because their eyes didn't have enough information about what was happening around them at any given moment in time!

Before you move on to the recommended exercises, take a simple test to see if you have serious issues in your inner ear, like a middle ear infection or bony deformity. These tests are usually be done by your GP or even an audiologist, and no special procedure is needed, so your insurance should cover it.

If your doctor says you don't need any medical treatment, you can move on to the exercises. They are pretty easy, and you can do them at home while sitting or lying down - or anywhere else you feel comfortable enough to concentrate on the exercises without distractions. The improvement time varies depending upon how well you focus on the task at hand, but most people who practice about 10 minutes a day for four-five days per week feel better within months.

Here are the exercises to start with.

1. Eye movement exercise: side to side

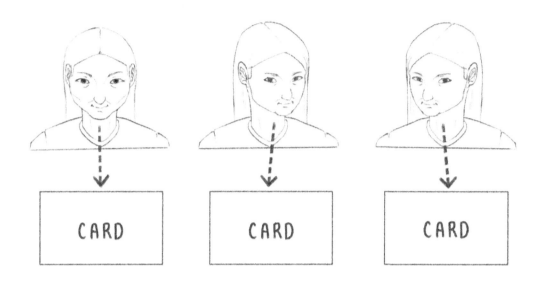

To perform this exercise, take a business card and hold it about 12 inches from your eyes. Look at it straight on without moving your head or body (you can also use an object like a pen or pencil). Make sure your eyes are relaxed and not squinting.

Now slowly move your head from side to side while keeping your gaze fixed on it. You'll notice that as you move your head, your gaze will naturally turn to the opposite direction and the card. Don't let your head turn too much - just enough (about 45 degrees) so that you feel like it's not straining your eyes when you move it from side to side and back again.

Once you've got the hang of it, try moving the card smoothly from side to side without moving your head. Try moving it back and forth while looking straight ahead at something else, like a blank wall in front.

2. Eye movement exercises: up and down

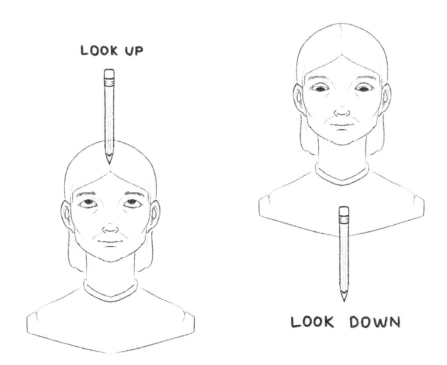

LOOK UP

LOOK DOWN

There are several ways of doing this exercise. One is looking up and down with a stick or pencil. You can do this very simple exercise anywhere and at any time. The idea is to look up at an object above you and then look down at your feet, making sure that your head doesn't move during the exercise.

To do this, lie on your back with your head on a pillow and your eyes looking up at the ceiling. Hold a stick (or pen) at eye level and move it up and down in front of your eyes about 50 cm away from you (the distance should be the same for all exercises).

Keep your head still, but move only your eyes to follow the movement of the stick. Make sure that you do not look at the tip of the stick, but keep your gaze fixed on its center, which will help to prevent eye strain or fatigue.

You can also do this exercise sitting up. Another variation is to move the pencil up and down, then side to side, and then obliquely to make an x. These movements help in exercising the six eye muscles that rotate the eyeball. This exercise is also beneficial for people suffering from droopy and unfocused eyes.

The next exercise is looking up and down without moving your head. As with the previous exercise, look up at an object above you and then down at your feet without moving your head or body in any way except looking up and down with your eyes alone. (This may be easier if you use a stick or pencil as described above.). This will help you move without any difficulty or pain in your neck, shoulders, or back muscles.

3. Head turning exercise

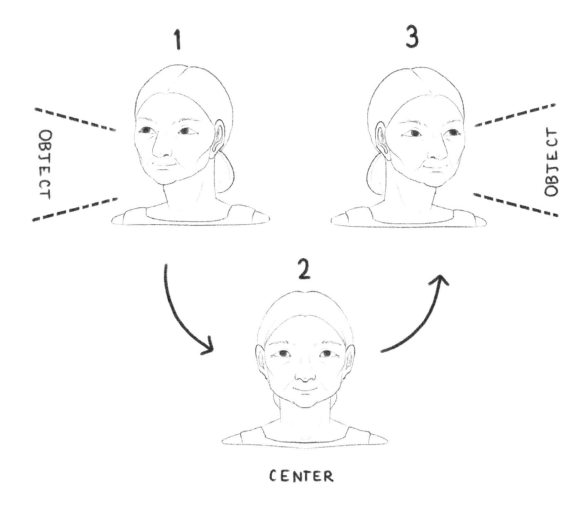

Head exercises are all about gaze stabilization. To start, set a clear target or point you will look at. You can only do the exercise if you can see clearly and the target doesn't move while your head is in motion. First, move your head to one side of the midline, keeping your eyes fixed on the target. Then move your head back to the center and repeat on the other side. Try to keep your head movements small (about 45°). Once you can do this, increase the speed of movement until you're moving quickly without missing the target or having it blur out of focus.

If you wear glasses, wear them while doing these exercises! They may cause symptoms of dizziness or nausea, but work through those symptoms, so they don't distract you from performing the exercise properly.

There are two versions of this exercise: one is sitting, and one is standing. Try practicing them both, especially the standing one. While you stand, keep your feet shoulder wide with a chair or wall close by for support. These exercises demand concentration; make sure there aren't any distractions around while you're doing them!

4. Spinning in a chair:

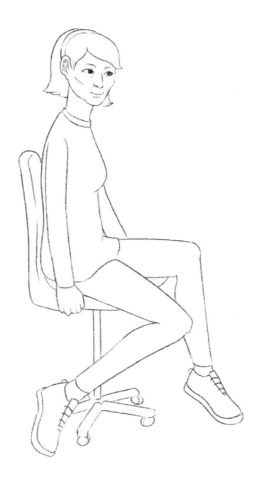

Spinning on a chair might seem like an odd exercise, but it really works out those little muscles inside our ears that help us stay balanced when standing upright! To do this, place a chair in the center of the room and sit in it. Place your hands beside you on the seat of the chair. Slowly lean back until you are sitting upright, with your back against the back of the chair. Your feet should be flat on the floor, shoulder-width apart. Now, swirl! Have fun while you are at it. You will feel dizzy at first, but after doing this for a few days, you will no longer be so dizzy by movements. But, as always, be safe while doing this, and don't go overboard.

5. Head/eyes turning vestibular exercise:

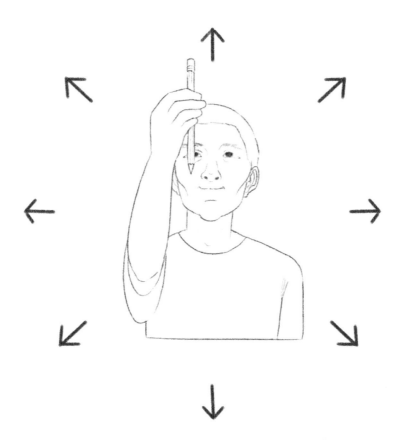

This exercise works with both your eyes and head. The coordination between the inner ear balance and your visual info is crucial for balance. So, it's good to exercise both senses together. To do this exercise, sit straight in a chair. Have a target; a handheld pencil would do. Now, move the pencil in a cross-motion. Your head/eyes should be moving in the same direction. So, while you are holding the target, keep your eyes fixed on it. Slowly move your hands and the pencil and turn your head and eyes in the same direction. Go up and down, then side to side and diagonally for several seconds.

There is no reason why you can't mix up the vestibular and balancing exercises. Here are some ideas to explore.

- Standing on one leg with your eyes closed helps improve balance by training the brain to rely on vision less often. It also improves muscle memory and strengthens muscles throughout your body.

- Bouncing on a trampoline or sitting on one while moving your body or limbs quickly in circles at different speeds. This helps improve vestibular system function by stimulating the inner ear while strengthening leg muscles at the same time.

- Sidestepping on an uneven surface like sand or grass. This helps improve your ability to step over obstacles without losing your balance. It also helps with balance on uneven surfaces such as sand or grass.

- Walking in a straight line without looking helps improve your ability to walk straight without having to look at anything in particular while it trains you to work with the feelings from vestibular organs.

It's important to consult a healthcare provider before trying these exercises. They can be done without equipment and are available for free online or from an audiologist. If you experience dizziness, stop the exercise immediately and seek medical attention. However, If you're suffering from only vestibular problems, then it might be worth trying some of these exercises. They are easy to do and should help with dizziness and poor balance. Consult a healthcare provider before trying the exercises and be sure to talk about what kind of exercise is right for you.

Key takeaway:

1. The vestibular organs in your inner ear are responsible for your sense of balance.

2. While you can't *see* these organs, you can exercise them with techniques suggested by doctors and experts.

3. Don't go overboard in exercising these, as many will exhaust your eye or make you feel dizzy. The idea is to slowly introduce your body to these so that you get less dizzy over time and the muscles and senses associated with balance get stronger.

Chapter 8: Lying Down Exercises

When it comes to staying healthy, many people focus on big exercises, like running or swimming. They are a bit difficult for seniors, but there are a number of easy exercises you can do at home without any equipment. These activities are especially helpful if you have limited mobility or can't stand up for long periods of time.

Lying down exercises can help improve strength and flexibility in your muscles, spine, and joints so you feel more mobile and less likely to experience pain or injury over time. These exercises are a group to be performed at home. They're suitable for people who have weak balance or who cannot perform some exercises due to pain.

Lying down exercises are also known as floor exercises or supine exercises, and they work every muscle in your body, from your arms to your hips. Lying down on the floor instead of standing up allows you to target different parts of the body without putting pressure on any specific joint or muscle group.

Lying exercises are beneficial to several groups of people, including:

- Seniors: in general, they have at least a slight difficulty moving around and often benefit from lying down because it's easier on their bodies. Lying also allows them to rest while keeping the blood flowing.

- People with back pain: Back pain is common among seniors, so they may find relief from this exercise if done regularly.

- People with knee pain: Knee pain can happen for many reasons, but one way to reduce your symptoms is by lying down and exercising in a way that rests the knees.

- People with hip pain: Hip problems affect nearly half of all adults over age 65 in the U.S., so it's important to learn how to keep them healthy by doing regular workouts!

One of the reasons that lying exercises are often used by the elderly and seniors is that they help to improve circulation, breathing, and flexibility by stimulating the inner organs. A lying exercise works on different meridians within your body and activates each organ as you breathe in the air into your lungs.

An example of a lying exercise is placing your feet together with your knees bent outwards. Your arms must stay relaxed at your sides with palms down towards the floor as if you were going to do pushups or sit-ups but without any pressure put on them at all!

There are many advantages of lying exercises for seniors:

- Lying on the floor is a good way to strengthen the back and abdominal muscles. You don't need to worry about whether your pose is right.

- It's easy for people with back pain to lie on their backs and lift up their legs or arms because this position doesn't put any pressure on their spines. Lying in this position also helps reduce inflammation in injured parts of the body, such as the neck or shoulders, after surgery.

- People with arthritis may find it difficult to stand up straight because they have trouble bending forward due to pain in their joints; however, leaning over while lying down isn't painful at all!

Here are some lying exercises to explore.

    1. Leg raise:

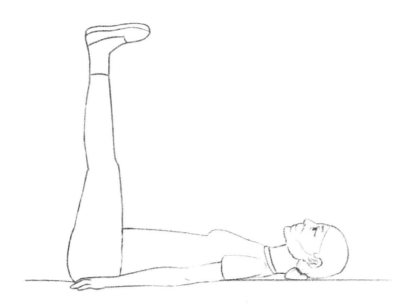

Lie back and bend your knees 90 degrees. Keep your palm and your feet on the floor. Lift both of your legs up, keeping them straight. Hold for 30 seconds, then slowly lower back down. Repeat ten times.

2. Supine leg raise:

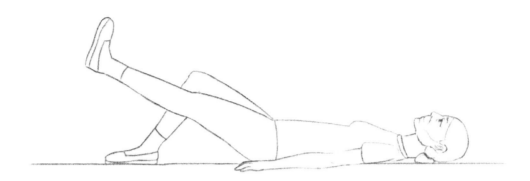

This exercise is great for core strength, hip flexor mobility, and lower back strength. To do this exercise, lie on your back. Keep your arms at the sides and your legs extended. Bend the knee of one leg. Slowly lift your other leg up to a 70-90 degree angle and hold for a few seconds. Lower them to the ground and repeat.

3. Butterfly crunch:

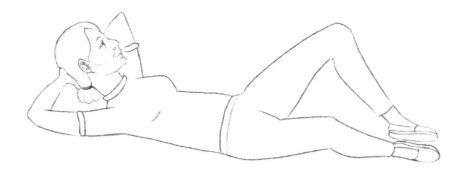

Lie on your back. Now, bend both of your knees and keep your arms at your sides while keeping the elbows bent. Bring your hands together above your head, clasping them together. Inhale and lift your head, shoulders, and upper back off the floor. At the same time, raise both legs off of the ground so they are perpendicular to the floor in a "V" shape (your thighs should be parallel). Hold this position for 2 seconds before lowering yourself down slowly again until you're flat on the ground once more. That's one rep!

4. Spinal twist:

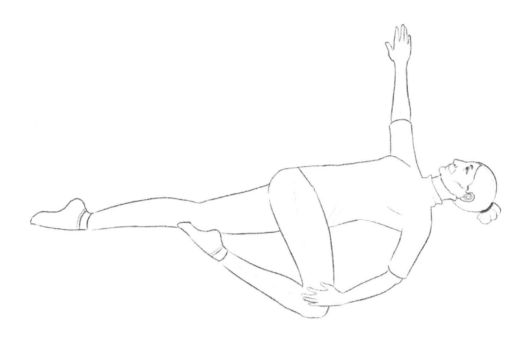

To do the spinal twist, lie on your back. Bend your knees and keep your feet flat on the ground. Stretch your arms out to the sides. Straighten one leg and turn to the side. Your bent knees should touch the ground. Now, hold your knees with your hand close to the ground. Then move your face to the opposite side and extend your arms wide.

Breathe deeply and hold for five minutes. If you're unable to hold it for that long, start with one minute and work up from there as you can. Do this exercise as often as possible during the day (ideally every few hours) for maximum benefit. You'll especially want to include this in your routine when pain flares up so that you don't have to make any sudden moves to relieve it—just stay put on the ground until it passes!

5. Lying glute:

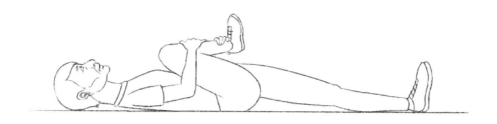

Lie on your back and keep the spine straight with your knees bent. Your feet must be planted flat on the floor. Now, lift one of the legs off of the ground, keeping it straight and parallel to the ceiling and straighten the other leg. Flex the raised leg's knee so it points toward your head. Squeeze your glutes as you lower your leg toward your chest by bending at the knee until they touch your chest and abdomen. Hold your knee with both hands and press. You should feel a good stretch in them. Return to starting position and repeat with the other leg.

If you have back pain and imbalance issues, this could be a good option for you! It's also helpful if you have tight glute muscles and gastritis.

6. Bicycle crunch

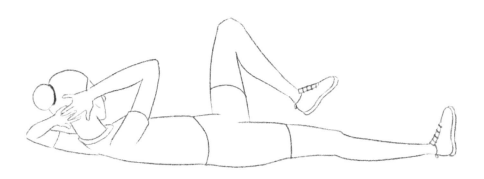

The bicycle crunch work on your abs. It's a variation of the traditional crunch, which mainly works the upper abs. Don't scoff at the sound of abs! Abs are great for balance! While doing this exercise, you will need to lie down on your back and keep both of your knees bent. Put one hand behind your head and bring one knee up to touch it with your other elbow (as if you were riding a bike). Then extend that arm out back while bringing the other knee up towards it until they meet again—this counts as one repetition! Repeat this process until you have completed 10-12 reps before switching sides.

Lying exercises are a great way to get a workout in and stay active.

You can do them at home or even while watching TV! If you feel like your body is getting tired from sitting all day, try these lying exercises out for size.

Key takeaways:

1. Lying down exercises are great for people who can't exercise due to spinal problems.

2. These exercises can be pretty demanding, so they can count as part of a complete workout.

Chapter 9: Advanced Balance Exercises

Balance can be a confusing topic. It refers to how well you can maintain your posture and body position when standing or walking. Balance is important because it helps prevent falls, which can cause serious injury or even death if they occur in certain situations (e.g., at night). Balance also allows us to engage in daily activities such as cooking, cleaning, or taking care of our loved ones without worrying about falling over.

The ability to maintain balance depends on several factors, including visual acuity (how clearly we see), proprioception (our awareness of where our body parts are located), the strength of muscles involved with movement (such as those supporting the spine), reaction time, and our sensory processing abilities.

When you're young, it's easy to balance on your feet and do simple movements like running or jumping. But when we get older, the concept of balance is a tough one to figure out. One minute, you're fine: you can stand up straight without any problems at all. The next minute, you're stumbling around. Even after a while, it is difficult to understand if you have gained enough balance from the exercises of previous chapters to attempt the harder ones.

In this chapter, we'll look at all these questions (and more) so you can gain an understanding of whether or not advanced balance exercises are right for you.

Advanced balance exercises are exercises designed to improve your balance and increase muscle strength and functional fitness. While they may sound intimidating, advanced exercises don't need to be difficult. As you get stronger and more confident in your abilities, these exercises will become easier as well! The key is finding an exercise that challenges you enough so that it's not too easy but still feels doable.

For example, a beginner might try a basic squat while holding onto your chair with both hands or keep your arms out straight in front for balance; an advanced version could be the same thing with one arm behind the back or both arms held out sideways like airplane wings (but not actually moving).

So, when should you do them?

You should do these exercises when you feel the most stable. If you are feeling dizzy or have a headache, it might be best to wait until the symptoms disappear before doing these exercises. When it comes to doing balance exercises, there are a few risks to keep in mind. When you have less control over your balance, don't do these exercises. If you already have health problems or feel dizzy or nauseous, check with your doctor before starting a new workout.

If you feel any of the below symptoms while doing these exercises, stop immediately and lie down.

- feeling light-headed or faint

- nausea or extreme dizziness

- confusion

Balance exercises for seniors are an excellent way to improve your overall health and reduce the risk of falls, injuries, and other injuries.

Here are some exercises to try at home.

1. Simple balance poses

Balance poses are excellent for improving balance because they help you focus on your body and not the environment around you. When we fall, we usually have a bit of tunnel vision and focus on the floor or other objects in front of us. In contrast, focusing on your body will help improve your sense of balance by helping prevent swaying.

Here are some ways to do a balance pose:

- Standing with feet together, press your palms together in front of the chest while inhaling deeply through the nose (as if meditating). Hold this position for five breaths before exhaling slowly through pursed lips. Repeat three times before switching sides.

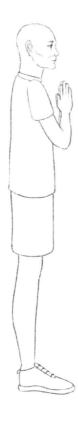

- Place one foot a few steps away from another as if making a lunge but with both feet firmly planted on the ground; hold onto something sturdy such as a countertop or chair back if needed. Bend the knees slightly while keeping shoulders straight as possible, raise the arms above head with your palms facing each other, and look straight ahead without turning head while maintaining this position for five breaths before repeating on the opposite side - again holding onto something sturdy if needed.

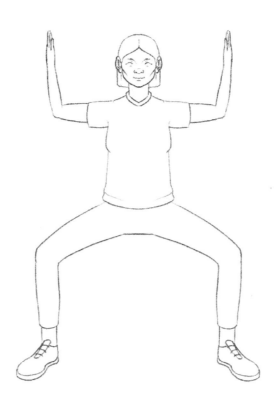

2. Flamingo stands balancing exercise:

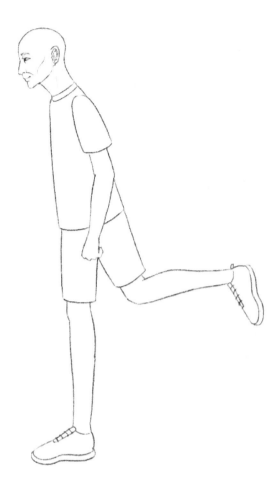

Stand on an exercise mat with your feet shoulder-width apart and your arms at your sides. Bend your knees and squat down until your thighs are parallel to the floor. Keep your back straight, chin up and chest out. Then stand again by pushing against the floor with the balls of your feet while contracting the muscles in front of you (quadriceps).

If you can't do this at first, try to do half of it. Stand on one foot. Now, bend the knee of your other leg at ninety degrees and keep it raised in the air. You will need to lean forward a bit to keep balance. As flamingoes stand like this for hours, this is called the flamingo pose.

3. Squat:

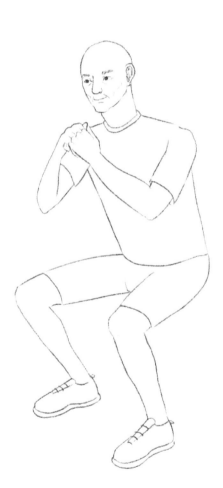

Stand with your feet hip-width apart with your hands on your hips. Keep your core tight and shoulders back as you lower down into a deep squat, bending your knees as if sitting in a chair. Pause when your thighs are parallel to the floor (or just below), then press back up. Keep your weight in your heels and push through the floor with your toes to return to starting position.

Make sure that you're not leaning too far forward or backward as you go down or up—it's easy to lose balance with this move! It's also helpful to hold on to something sturdy, if possible.

Try making this move five times each day. Rest for about 30 seconds between sets; aim for 3-5 total sets per workout session. This is a tried and true exercise for strengthening our legs and core muscles and improving overall balance.

4. Vrikshasana:

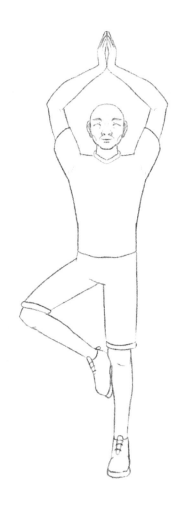

Vrikshasana, also known as tree pose, is a great balance exercise that can be practiced in either a standing or seated position. In this pose, you will have to balance on one leg. Now, bend your other leg and put the foot on your thigh. Then raise your arms overhead and put your palms and fingers of both hands together. Hold them up in namaste position. Hold for 10 seconds and switch sides.

This is a pretty advanced balance exercise, so have support beside you when you do it. For example, you can do this exercise against a wall.

5. Lateral hops:

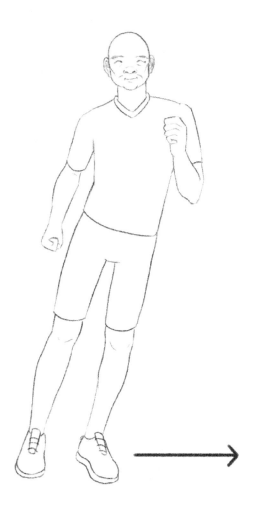

Lateral hops are a great exercise for improving balance and coordination. This low-impact exercise is easy to do and can be done indoors or outdoors. It can also be done in groups, which can improve social connections. To do this exercise, stand straight with your legs straight and feet a few inches apart. Keep your hands straight. Now, hop to your right side and while you do so, bend your left elbow and pull your hand up the side of your chest. Now, hop to your left and pull up your right hand to the side of your chest.

6. Eka Padasana:

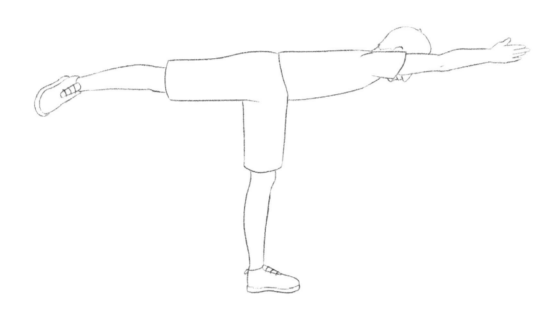

Eka padmasana is an advanced balance exercise that requires you to stand on one foot. This yoga asana strengthens your thighs, hips, and back muscles. It also improves your sense of balance, which can be helpful for seniors who are experiencing low bone density or recovering from a fall.

To do this exercise, stand straight with your feet shoulder wide. Now bend forward at your waist. While you do that, push one leg back up as well. Ideally, you should bend 45 degrees forward; your leg should be up by 45 degrees while you stand on one leg so, you make a triangle with your body.

7. Lunge:

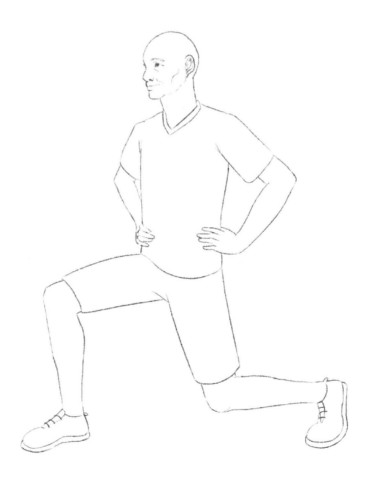

Lunges are an amazing exercise to build strength and balance. To do this exercise, stand with your feet together and hands on your hips. Take a step forward with your right foot, bending both knees so that your right thigh is parallel to the floor. Your left leg should be straight behind you. Keep your feet planted flat on the floor and keep your back straight. Hold this position for five seconds, then return to starting position with both legs together again. Repeat with the other leg as you advance. Make sure to be slow and step straight while you do this exercise.

In conclusion, if you are looking for a way to improve your balance and build muscle strength, then advanced exercises are the way to go. There are many different types of balance exercises that will help you get started. Ultimately, it all boils down to what type of exercise works best for each individual based on their personal needs and preferences.

Key takeaways:

1. Balancing exercises can be life-changing when done right.

2. You should be cautious while doing these exercises.

Chapter 10: Planning it out and Sticking to it

Exercise is a great way to stay healthy, but it's often hard to stick with it. It can take a lot of time and energy, plus there are so many other things you could be doing with your time! Fortunately, there are a lot of ways you can make exercise part of your life instead of something you have to push yourself through.

We all know that exercise is important for overall health. It improves our energy level and gives us more mental clarity, but sometimes it can be hard to motivate yourself to get moving: even to get your balance back. If you want to stick with a workout routine, it's helpful to plan your exercise schedule in advance so you stay on track. Planning makes sure that you have time (and a place) reserved for your workouts.

It also helps you find motivation. If you have planned activities for each day and week, it will be easier to stay focused on meeting those goals instead of falling back into old habits like sitting around watching TV or playing video games all day long! Your productivity will increase too. Planning ahead ensures that specific times are set aside specifically for working out; this means no excuses because everyone knows what needs doing when (and where). You'll start seeing results faster than ever before!

Plan your day

As you plan your day, keep in mind that you don't have to stick to an exercise schedule for the rest of your life. Instead, think about what types of exercise will help you meet your health goals. For example, if you want to gain balance, you don't have to exercise in the morning. Set a timer to exercise in the afternoon. If fitness isn't one of your top priorities right now but staying healthy is important, focus on ways that make sense for your life right now. Maybe it entails playing catch with your grandkids after dinner or tending your garden. Doing seated exercises amid nature is a good way to become more active without stressing too much about having a set workout routine.

Whatever exercises appeal strongly to you at this moment, in time they should be incorporated into your daily life; they'll keep things interesting while also improving both your mental and physical well-being!

Ditch the all-or-nothing attitude

When it comes to exercise, the all-or-nothing attitude can be a self-perpetuating cycle that sets you up for failure. One day you feel motivated and go out and stretch, but as soon as life gets busy or something comes up, all motivation goes out the window, and you don't go back again until another time when everything is perfect, and there's no excuse not to exercise.

But what if things never get perfect? What if life is always busy? That doesn't mean we have to stop exercising because we're not "perfect." The truth is that healthy habits aren't built overnight—they take time and consistency over months or even years before they become ingrained in your lifestyle.

By adopting an "all-or-nothing approach" to exercise (i.e., trying so hard that if you miss just one workout, it's easier NOT TO GO BACK), we end up setting ourselves up for failure because there will always be some reason why we couldn't make it happen that particular week/month/year. It may be watching your grandkids, too many conflicting appointments, friends who want us out with them instead...the list is endless.

Drink water

I know it sounds boring or irrelevant, but you should drink plenty of water regularly. Drink at least eight glasses of water a day. This is the minimum amount you need to stay hydrated and keep your body functioning properly, especially during exercise.

Also, make sure to drink before, during, and after exercise to replace fluid loss from your body. It's important to rehydrate quickly after physical activity as well as in preparation for it. If you wait too long before exercising again after sweating heavily, this can lead to dehydration later on in your workout session when you're already dehydrated (making it easier for muscles and joints to cramp up).

Get proper rest

In order to stay energized and motivated, it's important to give yourself enough time to rest. The recommended amount of sleep for adults is 7-9 hours per day. How do you know if you are getting enough sleep? If you feel fatigued during the day, have trouble focusing on tasks, or find yourself frequently yawning throughout the day (not just at night), it's probably a sign that your body needs some extra shut-eye.

Plan your meals accordingly

If you're planning to exercise, it would be a good idea to plan your meals accordingly. Eating healthy foods will not only help you feel better but it can also boost your energy levels so you can work out with ease.

The best way to eat for exercising is by having a balanced diet that includes protein and carbohydrates, fruits and vegetables, as well as healthy fats (olive oil). Avoid processed foods such as white bread and refined sugars because they won't provide the nutrients needed for strenuous exercise. Also, avoid sugary drinks like sodas or sports drinks before working out because these beverages contain high amounts of sugar, which can lead to an energy crash when it has been used up quickly in the body during prolonged physical activity.

****

FREE GIFT #2: E-BOOK "ANTI-INFLAMMATORY DIET FOR SENIORS"

Boost your balance and overall well-being by complementing your exercises with a diet that reduces inflammation. This e-book is designed to help you manage inflammation, which can impact your joints, muscles, and overall health.

To get your free copy, visit **bit.ly/Balance-audio** or scan the QR code with your phone camera if you prefer not to type. It's absolutely free.

This e-book is the perfect companion to your balance exercises, helping you achieve better health every day.

****

Get medical clearance

You should always get medical clearance before starting any new exercise program, especially if you have a medical condition. Your doctor or physical therapist can help you create an individualized exercise plan and determine what exercises are best for you based on your specific needs and abilities.

Choose activities that make you feel happy

Choosing activities that make you feel happy is the best way to stay motivated. Think about what makes you happy and then choose an exercise based on those feelings. For example, if the thought of walking makes you feel energized and confident, go ahead and go for a walk! If going out in the cold makes your muscles ache with exhaustion, don't go out! Exercise indoors in your cozy room instead; it's better for balance, anyway. You can also try looking at pictures of people doing things that make them look happy; this will put you in a good mood and remind you why it's important to keep exercising even when it doesn't seem like fun.

If possible, try finding ways to enjoy the exercises themselves instead of focusing on how much balance you are gaining or how many calories you're burning (if these your concerns). The key here is to remember that exercise should be enjoyable because it makes us feel great physically and mentally!

Make it a game

The best way to stick with your fitness plan is to make it a game. Make it a goal to see how long you can stay active or how many days in a row you can work out. Challenge yourself by competing against yourself and any friends who are also trying to get fit. If this sounds like something that could motivate you, try making a bet with someone else so that working out becomes part of the competition—and winning is an added bonus!

Mindfulness

Mindfulness exercises can help to remove negative thoughts and bring more mental balance. Mindfulness is a meditation practice that helps reduce stress and anxiety, as well as increase your sense of self-awareness. By practicing mindfulness, you will notice your thoughts and feelings without judging them as "good" or "bad." This skill allows you to let go of unhelpful thoughts while building a stronger sense of self-confidence. With time spent practicing mindfulness, even right before bedtime in the evening, you may find yourself sleeping better at night!

All in all, exercise is an important part of overall health. It can help you lose weight, feel happier, get better sleep, and reduce the risk of heart disease. So what's stopping you from exercising regularly? If you're like most people, it's time—or lack thereof. You have a busy schedule with family and other responsibilities, so finding enough time to exercise seems impossible at times. But if you're serious about improving your health and enjoying the benefits that follow (like losing weight), there are ways around the problem! If nothing else works for your schedule, try these quick tips:

- Exercise in short bursts throughout the day instead of one long workout session each week. For example: instead of going out for a run every Saturday morning from 8:00 am until 9:30 am (an hour-and-a-half), try doing 10 minutes here and there throughout the week—maybe before breakfast one day and before dinner another! If something comes up, you've got options!

Hopefully, this has been helpful in making you realize that it's possible to change your lifestyle and get healthy through exercise. The key takeaway is not to do too much of one thing; do instead, everything in moderation, so it works for you!

Key takeaway:

1. Make sure you're able to exercise regularly - at least three times a week. This doesn't mean you have to spend hours every day at the gym; even 10 minutes of activity on and off can add up over the course of a week. Whatever exercise plan you come up with will need to fit into your schedule three days out of seven.

2. Start small. The trick isn't so much to create the perfect exercise plan as it is to stick with it. Give yourself a simple plan and then follow through until it becomes second nature.

3. Set realistic goals. If you don't have time for a workout each morning before work, plan your workouts for a different time of day instead.

Chapter 11: 28-Day Challenge for Confident Balance

The journey to improving your balance and overall health starts with a well-structured plan. This 28-day workout plan is designed to guide you through short, daily exercises that will help you build strength, stability, and confidence in your movements. Each day's workout takes just five minutes, making it easy to incorporate into your routine, no matter how busy you are.

Why a 28-Day Plan?

A 28-day plan provides the consistency and structure necessary to establish lasting habits. Over the course of this month, you'll work through a variety of exercises designed to enhance your balance, targeting the muscles and movements that are most important for maintaining stability as we age. By committing to this plan, you'll not only see improvements in your physical capabilities but also gain greater confidence in your day-to-day activities.

The Structure of the Plan

This workout plan is divided into three progressive levels—

Beginner, Intermediate, and Advanced—spread across the full 28 days. Each week builds on the previous one, gradually increasing the challenge to match your growing strength and confidence. By the end of the month, you'll have completed a comprehensive balance training program that addresses all the key aspects of stability, from core strength to coordination and flexibility.

- **Week 1: Beginner** – In the first week, you'll focus on establishing a solid foundation with gentle exercises that are easy to perform. This week is perfect for those who are new to balance training or who want to start slow.

- **Week 2: Intermediate** – As you gain strength and confidence, the second week introduces more complex movements. These exercises will challenge your coordination and help you build upon the skills you developed in the first week.

- **Week 3 and 4: Advanced** – The final two weeks are designed to push you further. You'll encounter more challenging exercises that require greater control, strength, and endurance. By the end of this phase, you'll have significantly improved your balance and overall stability.

What to Do If You're Not Ready for More Challenging Workouts

It's important to listen to your body as you progress through this plan. If you find that some exercises in the later weeks are too difficult, don't hesitate to repeat the exercises from the previous week until you feel ready to move forward. Remember, it's better to progress slowly and safely than to rush and risk injury. Consistency is key, so even if you need to take extra time at a certain level, you'll still benefit from the regular practice.

What to Expect

Each daily workout is designed to be completed in just five minutes, making it easy to fit into your day. The exercises will help you improve flexibility, strengthen your core and legs, and enhance your overall balance.

As you work through this 28-day plan, be patient with yourself and stay committed. Progress might be gradual, but with each day, you're taking steps toward greater stability and confidence. By the end of this journey, you'll not only see improvements in your physical balance but also feel more secure in your daily movements.

Let's embark on this journey together, and take steady steps toward a more balanced and confident you!

****

FREE GIFT #3: 28-DAY BALANCE STRENGTHENING WORKOUTS TRACKER

As you embark on this journey to improve your balance and strength, I want to make it as easy as possible for you to stay committed and track your progress. That's why I've created a Printable 28-Day Balance Strengthening Workouts Tracker just for you.

This tracker will help you monitor your daily workouts, keep you motivated, and ensure you stick to your plan throughout the entire 28 days.

To get your tracker, visit **bit.ly/Balance-audio** and download it (along with other free bonuses). You can also scan the QR code with your phone camera if you prefer not to type. It's absolutely free.

Start your journey off right by using this tracker as your guide to staying on track and reaching your balance goals!

****

WEEK 1: BEGINNER

Day 1

1. **Seated Forward Punch (page 37)** – 1 minute
2. **Standing on One Leg (page 53)** – 30 seconds each leg
3. **Pelvic Tilt (page 39)** – 10 reps
4. **Seated Toe Raises (page 40)** – 10 reps
5. **Seated Forward Bend (page 43)** – 10 reps

Day 2

1. **Heel Lifts (page 57)** – 1 minute
2. **Balance Walk (page 67)** – 1 minute
3. **Seated Lateral Flexion (page 41)** – 10 reps each side
4. **Seated Hip Flexion (page 45)** – 10 reps each leg
5. **Single Leg Lift (page 79)** – 10 reps each leg

Day 3

1. **Heel Lifts (page 57)** – 10 reps
2. **High Knee Walk (page 70)** – 1 minute
3. **Seated Hip Abduction (page 47)** – 10 reps
4. **Seated Hip External Rotation (page 50)** – 10 reps each leg
5. **Plank (page 86)** – 20 seconds

Day 4

1. **Zigzag Walk (page 69)** – 1 minute
2. **Grapevine (page 72)** – 1 minute
3. **Seated Knee Tucks (page 84)** – 10 reps
4. **Seated Leg Lift (page 80)** – 10 reps each leg
5. **Modified Push-Up (page 82)** – 10 reps

Day 5

1. **Step-Up (page 73)** – 10 reps each leg
2. **Balance Beam (page 58)** – 1 minute
3. **Seated Bicycles (page 49)** – 10 reps each leg
4. **Lying Leg Raise (page 107)** – 10 reps each leg
5. **Head Turning Exercise (page 97)** – 10 reps each direction

Day 6

1. **Single Leg-Arm Stance (page 54)** – 10 reps each side
2. **Marching on the Spot (page 60)** – 1 minute
3. **Seated Pelvic Tilt (page 39)** – 10 reps
4. **Seated Hip Flexion (page 45)** – 10 reps each leg
5. **Side Step Walk (page 61)** – 10 steps each side

Day 7

1. **Spinning in a Chair (page 99)** – 1 minute
2. **Head/Eyes Turning Vestibular Exercise (page 100)** – 10 reps each direction
3. **Seated Hip Flexion (page 45)** – 10 reps each leg
4. **Seated Leg Lift (page 80)** – 10 reps each leg
5. **Standing on One Leg with Eyes Closed (page 53)** – 20 seconds each leg

WEEK 2: INTERMEDIATE

Day 8

1. **Seated Forward Punch (page 37)** – 1 minute
2. **Standing on One Leg (page 53)** – 40 seconds each leg
3. **Heel to Toe Walk (page 66)** – 1 minute
4. **Pelvic Tilt (page 39)** – 12 reps
5. **Seated Toe Raises (page 40)** – 12 reps

Day 9

1. **Rock the Boat (page 56)** – 1 minute
2. **Balance Walk (page 67)** – 1 minute
3. **Seated Lateral Flexion (page 41)** – 12 reps each side
4. **Seated Hip Flexion (page 45)** – 12 reps each leg
5. **Single Leg Lift (page 79)** – 12 reps each leg

Day 10

1. **Heel Lifts (page 57)** – 12 reps
2. **High Knee Walk (page 70)** – 1 minute
3. **Seated Hip Abduction (page 47)** – 12 reps
4. **Seated Forward Bend (page 43)** – 12 reps
5. **Plank (page 86)** – 30 seconds

Day 11

1. **Zigzag Walk (page 69)** – 1 minute
2. **Grapevine (page 72)** – 1 minute
3. **Seated Hip External Rotation (page 50)** – 12 reps each leg
4. **Mountain Climber (page 86)** – 12 reps each leg
5. **Modified Push-Up (page 82)** – 12 reps

Day 12

1. **Step-Up (page 73)** – 12 reps each leg
2. **Balance Beam (page 58)** – 1 minute
3. **Seated Knee Tucks (page 84)** – 12 reps
4. **Lying Leg Raise (page 107)** – 12 reps each leg
5. **Head Turning Exercise (page 97)** – 12 reps each direction

Day 13

1. **Single Leg-Arm Stance (page 54)** – 12 reps each side
2. **Marching on the Spot (page 60)** – 1 minute
3. **Seated Pelvic Tilt (page 39)** – 12 reps
4. **Seated Hip Flexion (page 45)** – 12 reps each leg
5. **Side Step Walk (page 61)** – 12 steps each side

Day 14

1. **Spinning in a Chair (page 99)** – 1 minute
2. **Head/Eyes Turning Vestibular Exercise (page 100)** – 12 reps each direction
3. **Seated Hip Flexion (page 45)** – 12 reps each leg
4. **Seated Leg Lift (page 80)** – 12 reps each leg
5. **Standing on One Leg with Eyes Closed (page 53)** – 30 seconds each leg

WEEK 3: ADVANCED

Day 15

1. **Seated Forward Punch (page 37)** – 1 minute
2. **Standing on One Leg (page 53)** – 50 seconds each leg
3. **Heel to Toe Walk (page 66)** – 1 minute
4. **Pelvic Tilt (page 39)** – 15 reps
5. **Seated Toe Raises (page 40)** – 15 reps

Day 16

1. **Rock the Boat (page 56)** – 1 minute
2. **Balance Walk (page 67)** – 1 minute
3. **Seated Lateral Flexion (page 41)** – 15 reps each side
4. **Seated Hip Flexion (page 45)** – 15 reps each leg
5. **Single Leg Lift (page 79)** – 15 reps each leg

Day 17

1. **Heel Lifts (page 57)** – 15 reps
2. **High Knee Walk (page 70)** – 1 minute
3. **Seated Hip Abduction (page 47)** – 15 reps
4. **Seated Forward Bend (page 43)** – 15 reps
5. **Plank (page 86)** – 40 seconds

Day 18

1. **Zigzag Walk (page 69)** – 1 minute
2. **Grapevine (page 72)** – 1 minute
3. **Seated Hip External Rotation (page 50)** – 15 reps each leg
4. **Mountain Climber (page 86)** – 15 reps each leg
5. **Modified Push-Up (page 82)** – 15 reps

Day 19

1. **Step-Up (page 73)** – 15 reps each leg
2. **Balance Beam (page 58)** – 1 minute
3. **Seated Knee Tucks (page 84)** – 15 reps
4. **Lying Leg Raise (page 107)** – 15 reps each leg
5. **Head Turning Exercise (page 97)** – 15 reps each direction

Day 20

1. **Single Leg-Arm Stance (page 54)** – 15 reps each side
2. **Marching on the Spot (page 60)** – 1 minute
3. **Seated Pelvic Tilt (page 39)** – 15 reps
4. **Seated Hip Flexion (page 45)** – 15 reps each leg
5. **Side Step Walk (page 61)** – 15 steps each side

Day 21

1. **Spinning in a Chair (page 99)** – 1 minute

2. **Head/Eyes Turning Vestibular Exercise (page 100)** – 15 reps each direction

3. **Seated Hip Flexion (page 45)** – 15 reps each leg

4. **Single Leg Balance with Eyes Closed (page 54)** – 40 seconds each leg

5. **Walking Lunge (page 125)** – 1 minute

WEEK 4: ADVANCED

Day 22

1. **Seated Forward Punch (page 37)** – 1 minute
2. **Standing on One Leg (page 53)** – 1 minute each leg
3. **Heel to Toe Walk (page 66)** – 1 minute
4. **Pelvic Tilt (page 39)** – 15 reps
5. **Seated Toe Raises (page 40)** – 15 reps

Day 23

1. **Rock the Boat (page 56)** – 1 minute
2. **Balance Walk (page 67)** – 1 minute
3. **Seated Lateral Flexion (page 41)** – 15 reps each side
4. **Seated Hip Flexion (page 45)** – 15 reps each leg
5. **Single Leg Lift (page 79)** – 15 reps each leg

Day 24

1. **Heel Lifts (page 57)** – 15 reps
2. **High Knee Walk (page 70)** – 1 minute
3. **Seated Hip Abduction (page 47)** – 15 reps
4. **Seated Forward Bend (page 43)** – 15 reps
5. **Plank (page 86)** – 50 seconds

Day 25

1. **Zigzag Walk (page 69)** – 1 minute
2. **Grapevine (page 72)** – 1 minute
3. **Seated Hip External Rotation (page 50)** – 15 reps each leg
4. **Mountain Climber (page 86)** – 15 reps each leg
5. **Modified Push-Up (page 82)** – 15 reps

Day 26

1. **Step-Up (page 73)** – 15 reps each leg
2. **Balance Beam (page 58)** – 1 minute
3. **Seated Knee Tucks (page 84)** – 15 reps
4. **Lying Leg Raise (page 107)** – 15 reps each leg
5. **Head Turning Exercise (page 97)** – 15 reps each direction

Day 27

1. **Single Leg-Arm Stance (page 54)** – 15 reps each side
2. **Marching on the Spot (page 60)** – 1 minute
3. **Seated Pelvic Tilt (page 39)** – 15 reps
4. **Seated Hip Flexion (page 45)** – 15 reps each leg
5. **Side Step Walk (page 61)** – 15 steps each side

Day 28

1. **Spinning in a Chair (page 99)** – 1 minute
2. **Head/Eyes Turning Vestibular Exercise (page 100)** – 15 reps each direction
3. **Seated Hip Flexion (page 45)** – 15 reps each leg
4. **Single Leg Balance with Eyes Closed (page 54)** – 50 seconds each leg
5. **Walking Lunge (page 125)** – 1 minute

****

FREE GIFT #4: BEYOND EXERCISE: SIMPLE STRATEGIES TO PREVENT FALLS

Congratulations on taking the first step towards better balance and stability! While balance exercises are a powerful tool, you can explore many other approaches to further enhance your safety and well-being.

That's why I've created an exclusive e-book just for you. This guide dives deep into natural remedies, supplements, home safety measures, cognitive training, and more.

To get your free copy, visit **bit.ly/Balance-audio** or scan the QR code with your phone. It's absolutely free and packed with valuable insights to help you stay steady on your feet.

I hope this extra resource gives you even more confidence as you work towards your balance goals!

****

WOULD YOU DO ME A FOVOR?

Thank you for reading this book.

I have a small favor to ask.

If you liked this book, would you mind taking a minute to write a blurb on Amazon?

I check all my reviews and love to get your feedback. That's the real pay for my work – knowing that I'm helping people.

To leave a quick review go to link:

amzn.to/3T1Q6zp

Or scan QR code with your camera:

Conclusion

Now that we have reached the end of the book, I hope you have picked up a few techniques for improving balance. As it was an in-depth book with lots of exercises and instructions, there are bound to be some that will suit you perfectly.

Exercises are a great tool when used correctly. It can help you lose weight, gain muscle, and get in shape. It hopefully has helped you regain your balance. Exercise is one of the most essential things in our lives; it keeps us healthy, active, and strong. But we all know that exercise has to be done right to have any effect.

Of note, there are a lot of ways to improve your balance. You can do it alone, with a friend or group. You can start slow and work your way up. You can even try different things that you've never tried before! Remember that exercise can be easy. It always works best when it is a part of your life. So if you want to get the most out of your workout sessions, make sure they're fun! If they aren't, you will be irregular, which means they'll stop being effective at helping your body grow stronger. So, be creative and make these workouts your own.

You have nothing to lose by trying something new, so go out there and get after it!

I hope that you've found this book to be a valuable resource. I know how important it is to understand that exercise can help improve your balance. We all know that practice is good for us, but sometimes it takes work to do it in a way that will make the most difference.

I'm excited to see what kind of impact this book has on you and your life. I know it's going to be amazing!

At **BODY YOU DESERVE Publishing**, we strongly believe that there are a thousand ways to improve your life and health. However, there is no single recipe suitable for everyone how to do that.

We think that the best way to receive your goals is the one you can stick to and our writers will do their best to provide simple, easy to follow, step by step and realistic instructions how to do that.

To discover our best books go to link:

https://amzn.to/40B5KmZ

Or scan QR code with your camera:

References

1. Lautenschlager, N. T., Cox, K., & Cyarto, E. V. (2012). The influence of exercise on brain aging and dementia. Biochimica et Biophysica Acta (BBA)-Molecular basis of disease, 1822(3), 474-481.

2. Kwak, H. B. (2013). Effects of aging and exercise training on apoptosis in the heart. Journal of exercise rehabilitation, 9(2), 212.

3. Quarta, M., Cromie, M., Chacon, R., Blonigan, J., Garcia, V., Akimenko, I., Rando, T. A. (2017). Bioengineered constructs combined with exercise enhance stem cell-mediated treatment of volumetric muscle loss. Nature communications, 8(1), 1-17.

4. Carapeto, P. V., & Aguayo-Mazzucato, C. (2021). Effects of exercise on cellular and tissue aging. Aging (Albany NY), 13(10), 14522.

5. Yoshimura, Y., Wakabayashi, H., Nagano, F., Bise, T., Shimazu, S., & Shiraishi, A. (2020). Chair-stand exercise improves post-stroke dysphagia. Geriatrics & Gerontology International, 20(10), 885-891.

6. Caetano, L. C., Pacheco, B. D., Samora, G. A., Teixeira-Salmela, L. F., & Scianni, A. A. (2020). Self-efficacy to engage in physical exercise and walking ability best predicted exercise adherence after stroke. Stroke research and treatment, 2020.

7. Pang, M. Y. C., Yang, L., Ouyang, H., Lam, F. M. H., Huang, M., & Jehu, D. A. (2018). Dual-task exercise reduces cognitive-motor interference in walking and falls after stroke: a randomized controlled study. Stroke, 49(12), 2990-2998.

8. Lichtenberg, T., von Stengel, S., Sieber, C., & Kemmler, W. (2019). The favorable effects of a high-intensity resistance training on sarcopenia in older community-dwelling men with osteosarcopenia: the randomized controlled FrOST study. Clinical interventions in aging, 14, 2173.

9. Sardeli, A. V., Tomeleri, C. M., Cyrino, E. S., Fernhall, B., Cavaglieri, C. R., & Chacon-Mikahil, M. P. T. (2018). Effect of resistance training on inflammatory markers of older adults: A meta-analysis. Experimental gerontology, 111, 188-196.

10. Li, F., Harmer, P., Fitzgerald, K., Eckstrom, E., Akers, L., Chou, L. S., Winters-Stone, K. (2018). Effectiveness of a therapeutic Tai Ji Quan intervention vs a multimodal exercise intervention to prevent falls among older adults at high risk of falling: a randomized clinical trial. JAMA Internal Medicine, 178(10), 1301-1310.

11. Sellami, M., Gasmi, M., Denham, J., Hayes, L. D., Stratton, J., & Bragazzi, N. (2018). Effects of acute and chronic exercise on immunological parameters in the elderly aged: can physical activity counteract the effects of aging? Frontiers in immunology, 9, 2187

Printed in Great Britain
by Amazon

46675702R00090